Your Medical Mind

Your Medical Mind

How to Decide What Is Right for You

JEROME GROOPMAN, MD, *and*

PAMELA HARTZBAND, MD

THE PENGUIN PRESS

New York

2011

THE PENGUIN PRESS
Published by the Penguin Group
Penguin Group (USA) Inc., 375 Hudson Street, • New York, New York 10014, U.S.A. •
Penguin Group (Canada), 90 Eglinton Avenue East, Suite 700, Toronto, Ontario,
Canada M4P 2Y3 (a division of Pearson Penguin Canada Inc.) • Penguin Books Ltd,
80 Strand, London WC2R 0RL, England • Penguin Ireland, 25 St. Stephen's Green,
Dublin 2, Ireland (a division of Penguin Books Ltd) • Penguin Books Australia Ltd,
250 Camberwell Road, Camberwell, Victoria 3124, Australia (a division of Pearson
Australia Group Pty Ltd) • Penguin Books India Pvt Ltd, 11 Community Centre,
Panchsheel Park, New Delhi – 110 017, India • Penguin Group (NZ), 67 Apollo Drive,
Rosedale, Auckland 0632, New Zealand (a division of Pearson New Zealand Ltd) •
Penguin Books (South Africa) (Pty) Ltd, 24 Sturdee Avenue, Rosebank,
Johannesburg 2196, South Africa

Penguin Books Ltd, Registered Offices:
80 Strand, London WC2R 0RL, England

First published in 2011 by The Penguin Press,
a member of Penguin Group (USA) Inc.

This book is based on the authors' interviews with patients who graciously shared
their medical histories with the assurance of confidentiality. All names, identifying
characteristics, and certain other details have been changed to protect their privacy.

LIBRARY OF CONGRESS CATALOGING IN PUBLICATION DATA
Groopman, Jerome E.
Your medical mind : how to decide what is right for you /
Jerome Groopman and Pamela Hartzband.
p. cm.
Includes bibliographical references and index.
ISBN 978-1-59420-311-4
1. Medicine—Decision making.   2. Patient participation.
3. Physician and patient.   I. Hartzband, Pamela.   II. Title.
R723.5.G753 2011
610—dc23
2011019808

Printed in the United States of America

1   3   5   7   9   10   8   6   4   2

DESIGNED BY AMANDA DEWEY

To Harry and Fran Hartzband, who taught us that a believer
and a doubter can share love and marriage and can
agree to disagree for more than six decades

i

Contents

Your Medical Mind

Introduction

We are drowning in information,
while starving for wisdom.

—E. O. Wilson

Every day, thousands of people consider whether or not they should take a medication or undergo a medical procedure. For some it's a question of prevention, how to stay healthy. Others must choose among different options for treating an illness. Making these decisions is harder than ever. There's certainly no lack of information—from doctors, the Internet, television, radio, magazines, and self-help books. Experts everywhere are telling you what to do. Some assert that you need more—more tests and more treatment. Others insist that you need less. How do you know what is right for you? The answer often lies not with the experts, but within you.

———

Dave Simon had been working for months to improve his serve. Recently retired, still trim and athletic, he was trying hard to bring his tennis game up to the next level. Now it was match point, and Dave was determined to win. He served wide and ran to the net, lunging to return a low volley. As his racket met the ball, he collapsed onto the cool clay of the court. He tried to get up but realized that his right arm and leg would not move. He heard his partner calling out to him, asking if he was okay. Dave had the words in his head to answer but found that he couldn't speak.

So this is what it means to have a stroke. My doctor warned me this could happen.

The door to the examining room clicked open and his cardiologist entered. Dave snapped out of his terrifying daydream. He was not on the tennis court, but in his cardiologist's office. He stretched his right arm and leg, reassuring himself that nothing had really happened.

"Good morning, Mr. Simon," the doctor said. "Have you had a chance to think more about the medicine? Are we going to start treatment today?"

On a routine checkup several weeks earlier, Dave's internist had found that his pulse was irregular. An electrocardiogram revealed that he had atrial fibrillation, a common abnormal heart rhythm. Dave was referred to a cardiologist, but his repeat EKG was normal. The cardiologist recommended that he wear a heart monitor throughout the day, which showed that he was still having episodes of the abnormal rhythm, even though he didn't realize they were happening. She explained that this condition could cause clots to form in Dave's heart; those clots might break off and go to his brain, causing a stroke. But the risk of stroke was low. There were medications that could help stop the clots from forming. But these drugs had serious potential side effects, primarily bleeding.

Dave was friendly with a neighbor who had been on such a drug. Several years ago, on a flight to Europe, his friend began to vomit massive amounts of blood. He almost died in the plane. The flight was diverted to Greenland, and the man, in shock, was rushed to the hospital. Emergency surgery saved his life.

Dave's mind veered back and forth between his chilling fantasy of a stroke and the image of his friend nearly bleeding to death. He looked at his cardiologist and replied, "I haven't decided yet."

Dave was caught in what psychologists call "decisional conflict," uncertain which option to choose. He knew the stakes were high and anticipated regretting either choice.

Susan Powell had already made her decision when we spoke with her. She wasn't going to take a statin drug for her high cholesterol.

Susan wasn't ignorant about high cholesterol and its consequences. Nor was she "in denial," as some physicians liked to put it. Fifty-one years old, she spent her days as a nurse's assistant caring for people of all ages and backgrounds with a variety of diseases from congestive heart failure to cancer. Her doctor had explained that high cholesterol levels could lead to heart disease and stroke and advised her to begin taking a statin pill. Susan was familiar with this type of drug, which is sold under brand names like Lipitor, Crestor, and Zocor. Some of the people she took care of were on it, and she had seen ads promoting these drugs on TV and in magazines.

"My father also had high cholesterol, and he died after a long and healthy life, without taking any medication." She told us that when her own health is at issue, she is the kind of patient who approaches medical treatment with skepticism. "I'm careful about what I put into my body, and I don't like medication," she said. "If I have a headache, I just deal with it; I don't immediately reach for Tylenol." Susan is a "doubter." You may see your own thinking in her, or she may remind you of a friend or family member.

Or you may take a very different approach to treatment, like Michelle Byrd. Michelle is an administrator at a university near Boston. She's in her fifties, too, she exercises every day, and she's proud that she can "power walk" two miles in less than twenty-nine minutes. Her college degree was in nutrition, and she is attentive to her diet. A routine checkup a few years ago revealed that she had mild high blood pressure. "I started taking medicine right then," Michelle told us. "I'm focused on doing the best I can for myself, and that means being proactive." Both her parents had hypertension, but neither had suffered any of its consequences like stroke, heart attack, or kidney disease. "And I don't want to either."

When Michelle Byrd began treatment, the first medication did not improve her blood pressure and a second drug caused side effects. She didn't hesitate to switch to yet another antihypertensive medication, and she's had no problem with this one.

Every morning and evening, Michelle checks her blood pressure at home and updates a chart of the results. "When there's a problem, I'll do everything I can to get as perfect a resolution as possible," she said. When we asked whether she was satisfied with her current systolic blood pressure in the low 120s, she paused and then answered, "I'm borderline okay with that." Then, after another pause: "Not really." She knows that 120 is viewed as a normal cutoff, but, she said, "I'd much rather be at 110." So she's asked her doctor to increase the dose of her current medication or add another treatment. He told her this wasn't necessary, but she still presses him for more. Michelle seeks to do the maximum. "That's the way I am. When I set a goal, that's it." Michelle is a "believer," certain that maximizing treatment is the best way to stay healthy.

Soon after we spoke with Susan Powell and Michelle Byrd, we met Alex Miller, who's also in his fifties. Alex is an accountant, a precise and organized man who spends his days crunching numbers. He has both high cholesterol (like Susan) and mild high blood pressure (like Michelle). While Susan Powell is convinced that taking a statin pill for her high cholesterol makes no sense, Alex Miller takes this medication every day, believing that it will help keep him healthy. So you might predict that Alex would be like Michelle Byrd in his approach to blood pressure readings above the normal range. But he decided that it doesn't make sense for him to take medication for high blood pressure.

Alex's cholesterol levels were consistent at each visit. But his blood pressure varied and was only somewhat elevated. After more than a year of discussion with his doctor, Alex reluctantly agreed to take a medication for his blood pressure. The pill had significant side effects. "I felt lousy, not myself at all," he said. His doctor tried to reassure him that the side effects would soon pass, and if they didn't, there were many other medications he could try. Unlike Michelle Byrd, who enthusiastically embraced a new drug after experiencing a side effect from a prior one, Alex Miller refused any more treatment.

Alex does not suffer from what some doctors call "health illiteracy"—a lack of understanding of the risks and benefits of treatment. His fluency with numbers allowed him to grasp the statistics his doctor showed him about high blood pressure and its potential consequences. But Alex had read on the Internet that some experts over the years had revised the definition of the normal range for blood pressure readings, designating what was once acceptable as now risky. "It's like they keep changing the goalposts," he said.

Alex knew not only about the consequences of hypertension itself, but about the many potential risks of treatment. "I wonder how many people actually look at the list of drug side effects, because if they did, they might not take any medication."

We asked him, "Does being so fully informed give you confidence in your decision or make you more worried?"

"Both," he replied.

Susan Powell and Michelle Byrd approach treatment choices quite differently. Susan is deeply doubtful about treatment and wants the minimum necessary, certain that "less is more." Michelle seeks maximal medical therapy, believing that by being "proactive," she is "ahead of the curve" in dealing with health issues. Alex Miller has elements of both approaches.

But isn't there a single indisputable right answer about treatment for each of them?

Despite many scientific advances, the unsettling reality is that much of medicine still exists within a gray zone where there is no black or white answer about when to treat and how to treat. Often, there are several differing approaches to treatment, each with its own risks and benefits. The best choice for an individual may be anything but simple or obvious.

People often explain their treatment choices by saying they do or don't feel "comfortable" taking a medication or undergoing a procedure. The discussion usually stops there. But what makes them "comfortable" or "uncomfortable" with one treatment or another, or no treatment at all? Where do these views about therapy come from? What are the forces inside and outside a patient's mind that shape that person's views? And will understanding those forces help patients to make better decisions?

After more than three decades of clinical practice, we did not have ready answers to these fundamental questions for our patients or for ourselves. Despite a rigorous education in medical school and residency training, then working in academic medical centers, we had never been taught how and why a patient might come to choose one treatment or another.

For answers, we turned first to medical decision analysis. This approach, drawn from economics and used by health care policy makers and insurance companies, contends that the experience of illness can be readily distilled into a number. These numbers should then be used to calculate the one "best" and therefore "rational" treatment choice. Difficult decisions become a matter of simple arithmetic. This kind of approach holds understandable appeal, but we found considerable research that shows it is based on false assumptions and fails to fulfill its promise.

As we continued to search for answers, the words of Sir William Osler, an eminent physician of the last century, came to mind. He famously said that when trying to unravel a complex medical diagnosis, you should listen carefully to the patient, because he is telling you the answer. So we turned for insight to people making choices about treatment.

We spoke at length with scores of patients of different ages, in different parts of the country, of different economic status, with different medical conditions, from various ethnic, racial, and religious groups. We asked them to tell their stories: when they first fell ill, how the diagnosis was made, what their physicians advised, and other information they considered when choosing their treatment. Often, we went back and spoke to them again, delving deeply into not only the clinical aspects of their experience, but the details of their lives—their families' attitudes about health and disease, whether friends or acquaintances had conditions that showed them the kinds of choices they might one day face, what knowledge they gained from their relationships, or their jobs, or their faith, that served them as guideposts. That journey into the minds of patients became this book. At each step along the way, as we listened to patients reflect, we gained more understanding. We then applied new research in psychology and cognitive science about decision making to their stories and began to answer the questions we raised.

It would be impossible to recount all the stories we heard, so we selected the ones that best illustrated specific influences on the medical decisions all of us make as patients. You will meet a teacher, a business consultant, a fitness trainer, an art dealer, a homemaker, a psychologist, a librarian, and many more. We're grateful to all these people for their openness and candor and their desire to share both their successes and failures in making their choices.

The book begins with decisions about problems that are not urgent and are often found on a routine checkup, like a high cholesterol level or a small rise in blood pressure, and then proceeds to conditions of greater urgency, like surgery, heart disease, and cancer. We ultimately reach the point where life itself hangs in the balance and choices may have to be made in a matter of moments or delegated to surrogates like family and physicians.

In each instance, we examine the powerful and often hidden influences outside and inside the patient's mind that can sway thinking and distort judgment. We saw that by unmasking these influences, it is possible to gain greater confidence and control over your medical decisions. That way, you can chart a clear path through all the conflicting advice and arrive at the right treatment for the right reasons.

One

Where Am I in the Numbers?

S usan Powell was one of the first patients we spoke with. We thought that starting with a common and seemingly simple choice—whether or not to take a statin drug for high cholesterol—would give us a simple answer about how people process information and arrive at their decisions. But Susan's decision was anything but simple.

S usan was up as usual at dawn. She made breakfast for her husband and her children and then checked the list of patients she would care for that day as a nurse's assistant. Late that afternoon she had a follow-up appointment with her new primary care doctor.

Susan had been healthy all her life. Like many women, her only contact with a doctor had been with the obstetrician/gynecologist who delivered her daughters and performed a yearly examination. But when Susan turned forty-five, she told us, "I decided the time had come for me to see a primary care doctor." Her gynecologist agreed and referred Susan to a young physician who practiced at a teaching hospital in Boston.

At her first appointment several weeks earlier, the doctor noted that while Susan ate healthy foods and led a physically active life, she was a bit overweight. Susan agreed to try to shed a few pounds. At the end of that first meeting, Susan had blood tests and at today's visit she would get the results.

"Everything looks good," the physician said, "except for a high cholesterol." The doctor paused. "You know there are two kinds of cholesterol, often called 'good' and 'bad.'"

Susan nodded.

"Your total cholesterol is 240, well above the cutoff of normal. Your good cholesterol, or HDL, is too low, only 37. And your bad cholesterol, or LDL, is too high at 179."

The doctor handed Susan a printout of her laboratory tests. "Since you're active and already follow a healthy diet, I think it's time for medication. Fortunately, we have good treatment for this. Here's a prescription," the doctor said, handing Susan a small green piece of paper with the name of a statin drug. "I'll see you again in a month, and we'll do blood tests then. I don't expect that you'll have any problems, but if you do, please let me know right away."

Susan took the prescription and put it in her purse.

Statins are among the most commonly prescribed medications in the world. In the United States alone, more than twenty-five million people take the drugs to lower their cholesterol. Cholesterol is a key factor in developing atherosclerosis, fatty deposits in arteries that can lead to heart attack and stroke. The first statin was discovered in 1972 by scientists in Japan. There are now more than a dozen varieties on the market. The drugs work by blocking an enzyme in the liver that makes cholesterol. Expert panels in the United States, Europe, and other countries have developed guidelines for prescribing statins based on the data from epidemiological studies as well as clinical trials assessing their effectiveness in preventing a heart attack.

Susan was familiar with the particular statin that the doctor had prescribed; many of her patients took the white pill that reminded her of a tiny football. Over the ensuing days, the doctor's prescription sat in her purse. On her way to church she passed the local pharmacy, but she didn't stop in to fill her new prescription.

At church that Sunday, Susan spotted an acquaintance of hers a few rows away. When the service was over, the woman, a little older than Susan, struggled to stand up. Her husband gripped her arm and slowly walked her to the adjoining room for the luncheon. The food was served buffet style, and the woman stayed seated while her husband brought lunch to her. When the meal was over, the woman's husband waved to Susan and beckoned her over. Other parishioners often came to Susan seeking advice with their medical problems.

"Are you okay?" Susan asked.

"Not really," the woman said. "My muscles ache terribly. And I don't know how long the pain will last."

She explained that she'd begun taking a statin a few months earlier. At first she felt fine, but over the past week she'd developed pain all over her body. Although her doctor had told her to stop taking the pill immediately, her muscles still hurt so much that she could hardly find a comfortable position, even in bed. And as Susan had seen, she couldn't get up from a chair or walk without help.

As Susan walked home from church on that bright winter afternoon, she thought about her father, Michael Powell. He was an independent thinker who questioned everything and never took anything at face value. Michael Powell also had high cholesterol, discovered when he was about the same age as Susan was now, not long after cholesterol was recognized as a risk factor for heart disease. "People take too many pills," he often told his children, and he never took any medication for his elevated cholesterol. He lived a long, full, and active life.

Susan returned to her doctor a month later.

"So, how are you doing on the medication?" the physician asked.

"I decided not to take it."

The doctor's face tightened in surprise and concern. "It's very important to take this medication," she said. "You really need it."

Susan Powell is hardly alone in her decision. Studies show that up to half of the people who are prescribed a statin for high cholesterol either never take it or stop taking it within a few months. Even in research studies where participants are carefully monitored with frequent visits and phone calls to ensure that they're taking their medication, people discontinue statins 25 to 35 percent of the time. This decision not to follow a specified treatment regimen, which some experts term "non-compliance" or "non-adherence," extends well beyond statins. Numerous surveys show that between 20 and 50 percent of patients with hypertension, diabetes, osteoporosis, or asthma don't follow the recommended regimen. A study of treatments for a variety of common illnesses conducted in 2006 for the National Community Pharmacists Association found that 31 percent of people never filled their prescription and another 29 percent stopped taking the medication before the supply ran out.

When we spoke to Susan five years later, we tried to delve deeply into why she chose not to fill the prescription. She certainly had seen the consequences of high cholesterol when caring for patients who had suffered a heart attack or stroke.

"I'm very much like my father," she said. "Everything he did, he did with gusto, always active. That's the kind of life I want to have. My father lived with a cholesterol level just like mine, and never took a pill." She paused, then added, "I believe that for some people a level of 240 is really dangerous. But for other people, like my family, that kind of number is not really abnormal, not dangerous."

Stories about people and the choices they make powerfully shape how all of us understand ourselves and the world we live in. This molding of our minds begins in childhood, when we listen to tales told by our parents and read storybooks at bedtime. As we grow up, we broaden our exposure to the experiences of colleagues, friends, and acquaintances. We also encounter a vast array of narratives from books, magazines, movies, TV, and the Internet. When we hear these tales, we try to locate ourselves in them. We imagine how we would experience life, what decisions we would make, in similar circumstances. Cognitive psychologists call the powerful influence of individual stories on our thinking an "availability bias." Certain tales and testimonials, especially those that are dramatic or unusual, become firmly imprinted in our minds; we remember them easily, and they are readily "available" to us when we ponder difficult choices in anxious moments.

As physicians, each of us has cared for patients for over three decades, and countless times we've heard people like Susan Powell recount how a family member, friend, or acquaintance decided to take a treatment and suffered its side effects—like the lady at church. Other times we've heard how someone they knew declined treatment and lived well into old age—like her father. We've also seen patients who came in requesting a particular medication or brand because of a testimonial from a friend with a similar problem.

Such stories can be reassuring or upsetting, but either way they profoundly sculpt preferences. Each vivid case becomes a mirror reflecting a potential future. Availability bias is perhaps the most powerful and prevalent force shaping how patients initially assess their options.

Of course, it was chance that Susan saw that woman in church. But if she hadn't, she would likely have gone on the Internet and found a similar tale from someone who felt fine and then suffered muscle pain, the most common side effect of statins, or someone else who developed liver toxicity and gastrointestinal upset, which are less common but also risks of taking statins. To be sure, seeing a person in front of you has a greater impact than hearing about side effects secondhand. But even secondhand stories affect the way people think.

We have also observed in our clinical practice that the stories a patient encounters, like that of the woman in church, may amplify preexisting mind-sets and biases. Susan is a doubter. "This was how I was raised," she told us. "This is how my husband is. And this is how we taught our children to deal with their health."

Other people may decline a statin medication because of the widely prevalent idea that natural is best. According to this concept, nature is wise, and the body does best on its own. Voltaire, who shared this view, asserted that "the art of medicine consists in amusing the patient while nature cures the disease."

Many people who subscribe to this idea believe they should rely on exercise and specific foods, like oat bran or red wine, or "natural" supplements to treat high cholesterol. They view medications as unnatural chemicals that pose unwarranted hazards. This mind-set can be termed a "naturalism" orientation or, in the language of cognitive science, a "naturalism bias." It is the firm belief that there exist smarter and safer natural ways to prevent and treat illness without resorting to synthetic solutions.

Gretchen Chapman, a professor of psychology at Rutgers University who has extensively studied how patients make decisions, illustrates such a bias with the following test: A person is asked whether he or she prefers a medication derived from a natural source like a plant or a chemically identical medication synthesized in a laboratory. People with a naturalism bias choose the compound from the plant even though it is indistinguishable from the one made in the lab.

Susan has never had any serious medical problems and feels good. "Every day, I count my blessings," she told us. She believes that she has much to lose by abandoning her skeptical approach and taking a medication. Her sense of well-being and independence; her pleasure in caring for her family and her patients; her joy in celebrating with her community at church—all of this, she fears, could be erased by a small white oval pill.

Susan is healthy, but even people who are not well will often hesitate to try a new therapy. The cliché "Better the devil you know than the one you don't" advises staying with the status quo as preferable to taking an action that could make life even worse. Psychologists call this "loss aversion." Research in cognitive science has shown that people experience loss more profoundly than gain. And one's aversion to loss is even more powerful when the potential gain is delayed or uncertain. In Susan's mind, her father would have gained nothing and only risked loss by taking medication.

Because all of us are deeply influenced by stories, we must remember that they represent individual events. Anecdotes are single cases, what researchers term "the n of 1." While the lives of people facing similar clinical dilemmas make a deep impression on us, they may or may not reflect the experience of the larger population. Stories can make real the risks and benefits of a treatment that might otherwise seem abstract—but they can also distort our vision by making the rare appear routine.

Statistics can often help put messages from stories into a larger context. Would Susan change her mind if she knew the statistics about high cholesterol and risk for cardiovascular disease that informed her doctor's advice?

Understanding statistics about the risks and benefits of a treatment is called "health literacy." It is an important skill because it enables us to grasp the scientific data about a therapy and make a more considered choice than we could possibly make using narratives alone. Susan's doctor put it like this: "Let me explain why this medicine is so important for your health. By taking a statin pill, you'll reduce your risk of a heart attack over the next ten years by as much as 30 percent."

Even with all her doubts, Susan found this an impressive number. But her thoughts returned to the woman at church. She asked, "What about the side effects?"

The doctor replied. "As I said before, I don't expect that you'll have any problems at this low dose. The risk of side effects is very small. At most, a few percent of people have muscle pain. And even if you get this side effect, it almost always reverses when you stop the treatment." The doctor trained her gaze on Susan. "The chance of side effects is nothing like the 30 percent benefit you get from taking the medication." Susan promised her doctor she'd give this new information serious thought.

Surveys show that more than 60 percent of people search the Web for medical information, and that number is increasing all the time. When Susan entered "cholesterol treatment" into Google, more than sixteen million entries popped up. She scanned the list from the top. Some hits were guidelines from medical societies; other sites were from pharmaceutical companies and hospitals; and still others were patient blogs.

Over the course of many months, Susan continued to search for information, reading everything she could about cholesterol. She found a government-sponsored link—a site from the United States Department of Health and Human Services. What caught her eye was "Health Information for the Public." There were numerous diseases listed, and Susan clicked on "Cholesterol." The link offered a "10-Year Heart Attack Risk Calculator," and she realized this was exactly what she wanted to know. Yes, her father was healthy all his life, but what was her own risk?

It was easy to input the requested information. She entered her age, total cholesterol number, and "good" cholesterol, HDL, from the laboratory sheet her doctor had handed her. No, she was not a smoker. Her blood pressure was fine, the upper number at 120. And she was on no medications. She then clicked on "Calculate Your 10-Year Risk" at the bottom of the display, and out popped the result. "Risk Score: 1%: Means 1 of 100 people with this level of risk will have a heart attack in the next 10 years."

Susan sat back and stared at the screen. This means that ninety-nine of one hundred people like me won't have a heart attack in the next ten years, she told herself. She started to feel much better.

Using the Web site, Susan had found a key number in health literacy, her risk for disease without treatment. Statin treatment will reduce Susan's risk for a heart attack by 30 percent. Now, let's figure out what this means.

Without treatment, Susan's risk for a heart attack was 1 in 100. If 1 in 100 women has a heart attack, that means 2 in 200 do, or 3 in 300. The statin treatment reduces risk by 30 percent, or about one-third. Let's apply that benefit to a group of 300 women like Susan, where 3 would have a heart attack without taking statins. If we treat

17

them all, we would prevent one heart attack—because we protect one-third of those 3. The other 2 women would still have a heart attack despite taking the medicine. The remaining 297 would not have had a heart attack even *without* the medication, so they wouldn't benefit from taking it.

This statistic comes as a surprise to many people. When you hear that a statin lowers Susan's risk by 30 percent, it sounds as if she is at 100 percent risk of suffering a heart attack if she doesn't take the medication. The calculation above yielded what is called the "number needed to treat," how many people must be treated to benefit one person in the group; for women like Susan, three hundred have to take a statin in order to help one person. By calculating the "number needed to treat," you can clearly grasp the impact of the drug for an individual.

A second key aspect of health literacy is knowing how the same information can be presented as either positive or negative. This way of changing how information is presented is known as "framing." We first framed the benefit of statin treatment by presenting it as a 30 percent reduction in risk. Seen this way, the benefit of taking statins appears very significant. But by reframing the benefit as the question "How many people do you need to treat to protect one person from a heart attack?" the benefit may seem relatively minor. Still, some people look at it this way: "If there is a chance I could be the one person out of three hundred who avoids a heart attack, then the statin is 100 percent effective for me."

"Decision aids" like the one Susan found on the Web site are designed to help people with a variety of medical conditions improve their health literacy. When you can interpret statistics accurately, you can merge science with stories and fit single anecdotes into the larger context of all people who are treated. Susan now knew the numbers relevant to her about statin treatment preventing a heart attack, and when we spoke, she considered whether she might be the one who would benefit. But she couldn't stop thinking about the woman at church. Susan's mind fixed on what she stood to lose.

The third component of health literacy is understanding the risks of a therapy. Susan's acquaintance at church had the most common side effect of statins: muscle pain due to inflammation. The medications less often result in liver toxicity and gastrointestinal upset with abdominal pain and nausea. As Susan's doctor told her, these side effects are seen in a "few percent" of patients. Statins cause muscle pain in 1 to 10 percent of people who take them. Some physicians believe you should drive down the LDL, or "bad" cholesterol, to very low levels by giving high doses of statins for greater protection against heart attack. But high-dose therapy with certain statins is more apt to affect the muscles. There is considerable controversy among experts over the risks and benefits of high doses of statins.

If we take into account both standard dose and high-dose statin treatment, we can accurately frame the side effects: The number affected is 1 to 10 out of 100. However, if we "flip" the frame, the number *without* any side effects is 90 to 99 out of 100, a much more reassuring statistic.

Susan continued to search on the government Web site. She read, "To find out what your risk score means and how to lower your risk for a heart attack, go to 'High Blood Cholesterol—What You Need to Know.'" She had all her numbers from the doctor on her desk. She again followed the steps on the screen and found that she fit into category four—low to moderate risk. The guideline said that her goal was to lower her bad LDL cholesterol to less than 160 by starting a "TLC" diet: eating healthy foods and exercising regularly. Susan read further. If the cholesterol didn't fall with diet and exercise, the guideline stated, "you may need medication."

Susan sat back in her chair and looked at the screen again. My diet is fine, she said to herself, and I'm getting plenty of exercise, on my feet all day long. She thought again about her chance for a heart attack and how treatment with medication might change that. "I decided the risk of a statin wasn't worth taking."

Howard Gardner, a professor of education at Harvard University, has written about how the same information can be presented in different ways. One way is numbers, and in the case of medicine, there are numbers about the risk for illness and about the benefits and risks of various therapies. This information can also be presented visually, often via a graph whose lines or bars convey the statistics. Last is stories, the narratives of people who faced these risks and benefits and how they fared. Gardner's research, along with that of many other educators and psychologists, shows that all of us respond most profoundly to stories; they echo in our minds and become imprinted in our memories. Ultimately, we want numbers and graphs to tell us a story—a story where we can imagine ourselves as the central character.

Advertisements for drugs may include statistics, but fundamentally these ads are designed to communicate a compelling tale. Over the weeks that followed her appointment with her physician, Susan Powell paid particular attention to ads for statins. Once she started looking for them, they seemed to be everywhere. The TV morning shows were punctuated with them; so was the evening news. Her magazines never failed to include at least a page or two that touted these drugs.

We had seen similar ads. And the more we thought about them, the more we realized that pharmaceutical companies understand a great deal about how people decide whether or not to take a medication. Drug advertisements are designed to overcome the psychological barriers to treatment that we witnessed in Susan's case, particularly loss aversion. They frame information about benefit in the most favorable fashion and exploit the power of availability bias using carefully crafted images and anecdotes.

The most vivid ads run on television. Many of these ads feature an ominous opening scene. In one, an older man is jogging while a voice-over soberly states that an elevated cholesterol level can lead to a heart attack. Next the viewer sees an avuncular physician prescribing a statin medication and the older gentleman nodding with a thankful smile. Then the mood becomes warm and bright, as the man (now presumably on the medication) is surrounded by his family at a birthday party. The camera focuses on the cake and lighted candles and the applause of wife, children, and grandchildren as the man blows out the flames with a strong, healthy breath. The implicit message of this story is that the man's rich, full life is sustained by the pill. Only when the viewer's attention is fixed upon the joyful birthday scene does a quiet voice list the drug's various side effects.

However, Susan focused on the side effects that were mentioned, undistracted by the positive images on the screen. "My daughter and I watched an ad together, and then afterward we just went back and forth with the side effects: muscle pain, stomach upset, liver damage. It's no wonder they try to distract you."

Advertising of prescription drugs directly to consumers is often justified as serving an educational purpose. Proponents claim that advertisements raise public awareness about health conditions and encourage patients to participate actively in their own care by learning about useful therapies and asking their physicians about treatments that may help them. In 2009, some $5 billion was spent on such drug ads, more than twice the total budget of the Food and Drug Administration (FDA).

A team of researchers from the University of California Medical Center at Los Angeles and other medical centers studied prescription drug ads broadcast on national networks. They selected commercials that aired during prime-time shows from eight to eleven p.m. as well as the evening news. The researchers found that the average American TV viewer sees over a thousand prescription drug ads in the space of a year. That's sixteen hours all told—much more time than the average person spends with his or her primary care physician.

The study concluded that the large majority of TV ads fail to fulfill an educational purpose. There was not sufficient information about the causes of the health problem, how common it is among different patient groups, who might actually benefit from the treatment, and how meaningful that benefit may be. Nonetheless, such drug advertisements clearly work, at least from the point of view of sales: Every $1,000 spent on advertising translated into twenty-four new prescriptions, according to an analysis by the House Energy and Commerce Committee.

Another illuminating study conducted by researchers at the Dartmouth Institute for Health Policy and Clinical Practice examined the impact of printed drug ads on patient preferences. The research trial involved more than five hundred adults. One group was given actual ads. A second group received the same ads, except that the brief summary at the end of the text was replaced by a "drug facts box." The box presented information in a clear, accessible fashion, similar to the way we recalculated the benefits and risks of a statin for Susan. Participants in the study came from across the United States and, except for a slightly higher number of women, largely reflected the country's demographic diversity. The ad for a statin showed a smiling woman who seemed to be about Susan's age walking briskly in the rain, holding an umbrella that protected her from the downpour. The image clearly communicated the message that statin therapy was a shield prudent people used to protect them—in this case, from a heart attack.

The results of the Dartmouth research are impressive. Nearly two-thirds of the group that saw the original ads and therefore relied on information framed by the drug company dramatically overestimated the benefits of the treatment. They believed it was ten times more effective than it actually was. But nearly three-quarters of the participants who saw the information in the drug facts box correctly assessed the actual benefits of the treatment.

Even more striking was another finding. When people were given readily understandable information about the statin's actual benefit in preventing future heart disease, nearly twice as many said they wouldn't take the drug in light of its side effects. This was an unexpected finding and contrary to conventional wisdom, the assumption that people do not act the way experts contend is "rational" because of a lack of clearly understandable information. Experts assumed that once a patient was "informed" accurately and completely about a medication, he or she would choose the treatment option that the experts saw as "best," in this case taking the medication. But in the Dartmouth study, this was not what happened. When given clearer information, the patients weighed the risks and benefits differently from the experts and were less likely to take the medication.

Loss aversion, the reluctance to risk side effects for what is perceived to be a small future benefit, becomes more powerful for many people in the setting of more understandable information. The Dartmouth research shows that Susan is not an outlier in declining statin therapy after learning all the numbers.

———

Not long after Susan saw the primary care physician, her employer changed the company's health insurance plan, and she had the option to find another doctor who accepted her new coverage. She chose Dr. Jacques Carter, who practices at our hospital. For the past four years, he has been her internist. He's a tall, broad-shouldered man in his early sixties, with a ready smile. He told us that he likes to begin with banter before raising the contentious issue of statin treatment with a patient like Susan.

"Gee, I think I see something that looks familiar," Carter said at her most recent visit.

Susan laughed.

"Your blood tests show that your cholesterol is still high." Carter looked squarely at Susan. "The level is now 280. I really think you need to be on medication." Using the same government calculator, her risk for a heart attack had risen to 2 percent, up from 1 percent. The number needed to treat was now 1 in 150.

"I'll work even harder on my diet," she replied.

"Keep working on it. But you know I'm not going to give up," Carter said.

Susan nodded. "And neither am I," she responded.

Shortly after their meeting, we spoke with Dr. Carter. "So often a patient's preference has nothing to do with education," he told us. "You are continuously surprised by people like Susan Powell. She works as a nurse's assistant and sees every possible complication of atherosclerosis and still won't take a statin."

When Susan had repeatedly declined to take a statin, her previous primary care doctor told her flatly that if patients don't follow her instructions, she can't care for them. When we spoke with Jacques Carter, he said he was familiar with this story and shook his head.

"That's just wrong. It's the old, paternalistic way of dealing with patients. Ultimately, you know, patients have final control of what goes on. And once a doctor realizes that—that patients don't have to take what you prescribe—then you realize that if you want them to do things you think will benefit them, you have to sit down and talk and come to an understanding. Caring for people is all about negotiation."

Jacques Carter grew up in North Carolina, the son of a plumber's assistant who couldn't advance in the trade because he was African American. Before going to medical school, Carter worked in Washington, D.C., for that city's Department of Health. His job was to improve sanitation, monitoring the sewer system, trash collection, and other community needs. In that job, "you had to learn how to talk to people," he explained. "You can't just tell them what to do. That's where I first became so aware of the importance of negotiation. People want to discuss why they do what they do."

The first time Carter meets with a patient, he doesn't expect him or her to immediately follow his advice. "You are putting a lot of stuff out there, lots of numbers about benefit and risk. But often people will say, 'No, I don't want to take that medicine. I just don't want that.' Or they say they're worried if it really is best for them. So, you bring them back in a month or two months, and then bring it up again. And still they say no. And then the third time when you raise the issue, you see that they are thinking about it more deeply.

"As a doctor, you are jockeying for position. It's not an efficient process. It's not like you just go, 'Boom, boom, boom, here is the prescription.' Because too often I've found a patient at that point will smile at you, take the prescription, put it in her pocket, and never take the medication."

When Susan Powell first met with Dr. Carter to discuss her cholesterol, she told him, "It's my body, and whatever I put in it, it's going to affect me. It's fine for you to advise me differently, to tell me that by not taking the statin pill this is what could happen over the short term or the long term, and how much damage might be done. That's fine. But remember that there are side effects. Everything from stomach pains to muscle damage. None of those things has ever happened to me."

As Susan found in her Web search, national guidelines recommend statin treatment for women like her if diet and exercise are not enough to lower her cholesterol. However, some experts question this recommendation and believe the benefits for any single patient do not clearly outweigh the risks. Dr. Carter, who has a master's degree in public health from Harvard University in addition to his MD from Georgetown University, is especially alert to the contrast between guidelines for groups and advice for individuals. "Taking care of individual patients requires you to think differently than when you are talking about entire populations," Carter said. It is much easier to grasp the impact of a pill that changes the risk of a heart attack from 1 percent to 0.7 percent when you're making recommendations for millions of people with high cholesterol rather than for Susan Powell alone. Framed as a public health issue, statin use may seem like an imperative. But when framed as a personal health issue, the benefits of taking statins may seem less compelling.

Dr. Carter told us that although he hoped otherwise, Susan Powell's condition might change in the future—and with it her point of view. She could develop a symptom related to her high cholesterol, like chest pain from coronary artery disease or dizziness from buildup of plaque in an artery to the brain. In effect, Carter was acknowledging how difficult it is for a patient who feels good to imagine a future illness. But short of developing symptoms, "she's not likely to get on the medicine." So, he continued, "in her case, I have to address everything else about her life that could be a cardiac risk factor. I keep close track of her blood pressure. I'm trying to get her to lose some more pounds, and even though she's quite active, encourage her to do a bit more exercise."

Carter will also keep telling her to take the drug "because I think that it may make a difference. But clearly there are people with cholesterol numbers as high as or even higher than hers who are well into their eighties and doing fine. She could live a long and happy life without the medication."

In this short and seemingly straightforward interchange between Susan Powell and Dr. Carter, there is much to learn. From the outset, Susan is the kind of person who wants to be sure that her doctor subscribes to the fundamental principle of patient autonomy. It is the patient who ultimately benefits from a treatment or suffers the consequences of its side effects, so ultimately it is the patient who should decide. As Susan indicated, this principle doesn't mean that she's always right or that the doctor shouldn't challenge her with a contrary point of view. In fact, during one of our interviews, she said bluntly, "I'm not afraid to be challenged. But when I lay out my position, I want to be understood."

Susan Powell has declined statin therapy for more than five years. Yet she told us, "If I had cancer, it would be different." That is, if she had an urgent and life-threatening problem like cancer, she wouldn't avoid treatment. Although she would opt for a treatment that minimized side effects if at all possible, her skeptical approach isn't enough to rule out radiation or chemotherapy. So Susan Powell's preferences about medication for elevated cholesterol do not reflect a rigid or fixed mind-set. Preferences about treatment turn out to be more fluid and flexible than many might imagine.

Susan told us a story about a friend of hers that illustrates how Susan herself might approach a cancer diagnosis. "My friend was told she needed surgery to remove a cancer in her throat and then chemotherapy." The friend told Susan that she didn't want to undergo the treatment. "I'm not a doctor, but family and people at church still often ask me for medical advice, since I work in the health field." Susan asked her friend, "What did you read about the treatment? What did the doctor tell you about the side effects? What are you willing to live with? What does it take to really deal with that particular condition?" Susan told her friend, "Look, the choice is yours. We're all going to die, but if there is the possibility to save your life, to give you the opportunity to live longer, even with all the side effects and problems, would you choose that?" Susan always couches her replies with, "This is my personal opinion. It's for you to choose." Her friend ultimately chose the treatment, and while it was very difficult for her, and she is left with impaired speech and difficulty eating certain foods, she's happy with her choice.

As we've seen, Susan's decision was not simple. She had to weigh information about benefit and risk that can be framed in various ways. Then she had to wrestle with the potent influence of personal stories as well as the power of loss aversion and her doubter orientation.

After we spoke with Susan, we started to think about our own experiences with medical treatment, both as physicians and as patients. During many morning walks around our neighborhood, we had animated conversations about our own mind-sets, values, and preferences.

We realized that each of us had started our careers with a different conception of medical care. The old saw "Opposites attract" applied to us. One of us, like Michelle Byrd, believed in being as proactive as possible. The other, like Susan Powell, was deeply wary of overtreatment. We found this odd, since there was little difference between the medical schools where we'd trained and none between the hospitals where we'd worked.

We concluded that to better understand why patients choose as they do, we needed to first understand the origins of our own views about treatment and how they evolved.

Two

Believers and Doubters

One of the first skills that we learned as medical students was to "take a history" from a patient. We were taught to follow a structured sequence, first exploring when symptoms began, how they may have changed over time, what may have made them better or worse. Then we would ask the patient about his prior illnesses and therapies and the health of his family—grandparents, parents, and siblings. In the last part of the interview, we would ask about current and prior habits like cigarette smoking and alcohol consumption, as well as lifestyle, including exercise, diet, marital or other relationships, and the person's type of work. All of this information gives doctors a clearer understanding of the nature and origin of the current condition and how it fits into the patient's life as a whole.

We thought about unraveling preferences about treatment in much the same way we take a medical history. Family is the starting place for many people's attitudes and values, and medicine is no exception. Around the kitchen table, during summer vacations, when holidays are celebrated, and the myriad other times families gather, people talk about health and illness, learning about the choices their relatives have made and forming a foundation for their own thinking. So we decided to consider the "family history" first. We then would explore previous experiences in navigating earlier medical problems, the "past medical history." Next we would focus on knowledge about others who suffered similar maladies—friends, stories on television or in magazines, testimonials on the Internet—this was the "social history." By focusing on these three elements, we hoped to create a framework that would help us to better understand preferences about treatment and how they came to be.

We decided to test this approach on ourselves to see what we would learn.

[Jerry's Narrative]

"Cholesterol."

I was eleven years old and had never heard the word before. It was 1963, and suddenly cholesterol seemed to be everywhere. Cholesterol was repeatedly invoked by my parents at the kitchen table. Reports filled TV broadcasts and the newspapers. Doctors were checking it, and the men in my neighborhood compared their results. My father's level was high—exactly how high I don't recall, but the number became an obsession in the family. Overnight, our cuisine changed. Egg yolks disappeared. Gone was the sweet butter. Hot pastrami sandwiches were restricted to special occasions and even then only extra-lean meat; the delicious edges of fat were removed.

A year after cholesterol was banished from our kitchen, the surgeon general of the United States released his report on the association of cigarette smoking with cancer. During the Second World War, my father joined the United States Army, was sent to France, and there became a smoker like so many of his fellow soldiers. My mother, a young beauty in the neighborhood when my father left for war, had grown into a mature woman. As a sign of independence and sophistication, she too started to smoke. Both my father and my mother quit cold turkey in response to the government report. Then my father's blood pressure was found to be high. The salt shaker, once omnipresent at meals, now stayed out of sight. So did those wonderful dishes of herring cured in brine. Our family doctor gave my father a diuretic, a water pill, but this seemed to have scant effect on lowering his numbers.

Despite the drastic changes, our home was anything but dour. My parents had a lively sense of humor. My mother loved to laugh in response to my father's wordplay. He delighted in funny phrases, many of them expressions only partly translated from the original Yiddish into English. One of his favorites was, *"Es tieten bahnkis,"* the last word having a silly dual-syllable resonance: *bahn-kis*. The loose translation is, "It's as effective as cupping," and the meaning was, "It's useless." Cupping was an Eastern European folk remedy. You put a small amount of alcohol in the bottom of a glass cup with a wick, lit it, and then placed the hot cup on the ailing person's back. The idea was that the heat and vacuum from the evaporated alcohol would suck out the harmful humors that led to the illness. This method was a throwback to an outmoded medical belief that diseases were caused by an imbalance of various humors (that is, fluids like phlegm, blood, and bile) in the body. *Bahnkis* was one of many specious beliefs about what caused illness and the ridiculous ways to remedy it. In my house, naturalism was seen as part of this primitive past, practiced by village shamans and benighted elders. Modern science had replaced this naive reliance on nature and the body's ability to heal itself. Not surprisingly, medical researchers stood on a pedestal in my home. We considered Jonas Salk and Albert Sabin to be as heroic in their battles against polio as Franklin Roosevelt and Winston Churchill had been in the war that brought my father to France.

In college, I was drawn to the intellectual dimension of human biology, how cells and tissues and organs work through DNA and RNA and proteins. A life could be devoted to figuring out why these essential components go awry and result in disease. I was in part imagining myself as the medical sleuth, the clinical detective on the hunt for the hidden perpetrator that threatened the life of a patient. And then I encountered illness, not in a textbook or classroom, but in my family.

On a warm spring night in 1974, I saw my father struggle to live. At the time, I was in my second year of medical school at the Columbia University College of Physicians and Surgeons in Manhattan. My family lived in Queens in a neighborhood of small homes and apartments not far from a local hospital. I had been asleep when my mother called and told me in a frantic voice that my father had had a heart attack, and she had taken him to that hospital.

In less than an hour, I was at his side. The hospital was a small four-story structure made of brick painted white. My father was in the emergency room. There were six beds, each separated by a flimsy curtain. A middle-aged physician unknown to me or my mother was on call that night. My mother and I gripped each other in silence as we watched my father gasp for air. He was bolt upright in bed, his hair in disarray, matted down by sweat. His warm, ruddy complexion had turned an ivory white, and his eyes were rolled upward. An intravenous line had been inserted in his arm, and from a catheter above his collarbone, the doctor was removing pints of bright red blood.

"You should leave now," the doctor said.

My mother and I retired to a small waiting area next to the ER.

I looked at the clock and saw the hour hand approach two. Less than thirty minutes later, the doctor came out with a grim face and told us that Seymour Groopman had died. He was fifty-five years old and the center of my life.

My father's death cast a long shadow over my life and the life of my family. He was never far from my mind during my internship and residency training at the Massachusetts General Hospital (MGH). There, other men in their fifties, who also smoked, had put on weight, and had high blood pressure, came "crashing," as the hospital jargon put it, into the emergency room, paramedics pumping on their chests. At those moments, I realized how my father had received dismal care in Queens. I didn't have all the details about my father's treatment, but I learned at MGH that removing pints of blood as a way to "unload" the burden on a failing heart was a dated and discarded approach. And though my father struggled to breathe as fluid built up in his lungs, causing pulmonary edema, he wasn't intubated and placed on a ventilator, which would have assured delivery of oxygen to his heart and other vital organs. At MGH, modern interventions were rapidly marshaled to try to save a stricken man's life. After doctors placed a tube in the trachea to supply oxygen, powerful medications called pressors were given to prevent the circulatory system from collapsing. When these measures were not enough, a counterpulsation balloon pump was placed into the aorta, acting as a surrogate heart to move blood through the body and sustain life. And if this proved insufficient, a team of cardiac surgeons would take the patient to the operating room to try to open his coronary vessels. Each time the ER team, working with cardiologists and cardiac surgeons, saved the life of a heart attack victim, I rejoiced.

But the joy soon gave way to sadness. I could not unhinge my mind from the fact that the doctor in the Queens hospital had glaring gaps in knowledge and ability. If my father had been given proper care, perhaps he could have been saved. Perhaps not. But if not, there would be no searing sense of regret.

So the culture of my upbringing and the trauma of my father's death made me a believer in modern medicine, its power and its promise. After my residency at MGH, I sought like-minded physicians with whom to train and work. I considered but ultimately did not choose cardiology. Rather, I entered a field that was less advanced at the time: oncology. The understanding of cancer in the 1970s was primitive. But soon came the DNA revolution with molecular biology. Mapping genes pinpointed the mutations that transformed a healthy cell into a cancerous one. Cancer cells then grow without restraint and spread from the tissue of origin to invade and destroy other parts of the body. I decided I would dedicate myself in the laboratory and the clinic and prove that even under the most dire circumstances of malignancy, science had answers. UCLA Medical Center offered one of the most intensive training programs in the nation, and I went there.

My mentors at UCLA were maximalists in treatment, firmly committed to doing everything all the time. And that determination when treating life-threatening illnesses often made sense. UCLA was home to one of the country's first bone marrow transplantation centers. During my training, I was part of the team transplanting patients with fatal blood diseases like leukemia. Bone marrow transplantation was an attempt at medical resurrection; patients were brought to the brink of death and then given blood stem cells to try to rescue them. The first years of marrow transplant were grim: All the patients suffered terrible toxicity from the treatment, and very few survived. Yet Dr. E. Donnall Thomas in Seattle and others were believers—like Salk and Sabin, who believed it was possible to eradicate polio. Belief is necessary for progress against deadly and disabling diseases. Don Thomas persisted with stubborn determination in advancing the therapy of marrow transplantation. The treatment was refined, and while still fraught with complications, it ultimately was proven curative for a wide variety of blood-related cancers. Thomas was awarded the Nobel Prize in 1990 in recognition of the countless lives this procedure had saved.

These kinds of successes shaped my approach to cancer treatment. I was drawn to what Stephen J. Gould—the Harvard biologist who developed mesothelioma, a rare and usually lethal malignancy, and lived twenty years after the diagnosis—called the "tail of the curve." In his essay "The Median Isn't the Message," Gould discussed how, as an evolutionary biologist, he understood the remarkable variability of all living beings and a similar diversity in how disease and its treatment play out in any individual. That view, drawn from his life's work in research, gave Gould the hope that he might be in that small but real fraction of survivors. Gould also raised the prospect that if he survived long enough, new treatments might be developed to improve the outcome of even the most desperate diseases like his. I saw Gould's hope in experimental treatments realized during my training as a fellow in hematology and oncology.

A high school teacher in his thirties, the son of Mexican American immigrants with a devoted wife and two young daughters, came to UCLA for an experimental therapy for his testicular cancer. With standard treatments the malignancy had spread widely, his lungs filled with metastases the size of golf balls. At the time, researchers were testing a new anticancer treatment, cisplatinum, a drug based on that metal. The teacher knew what he was facing, so despite the risk of toxicity of the new drug, including kidney damage, neuropathy, and hearing loss, he readily signed the informed consent document.

Three months later, the man's cancer was completely gone. I had witnessed what is often termed "a medical miracle," a moment when desperate hope is fulfilled against all odds. The story of that success is now widely known, largely because of Lance Armstrong, whose testicular cancer had spread not only to his lungs but also to his brain and who subsequently went into remission and won seven Tours de France. There are such moments when the dream of a new therapy that restores life becomes reality. In the early 1980s, when I first became a staff physician at UCLA, I saw people with AIDS die terrible deaths in months; a decade later, with the discovery of new drugs, the protease inhibitors, the death rate plummeted and lives were restored. Many children with neuroblastoma and adults with lymphoma now can go into remission with breakthrough therapies like monoclonal antibodies that did not exist when I started my training. To be sure, scientific advances are unpredictable. Many fail, but a few succeed. For me, that uncertainty was a basis for treating patients with severe illness in an intensive and sustained way, struggling to keep them alive until better therapies might arrive.

Every day after work, a group of hematologists and oncologists gathered near the UCLA Medical Center dressed not in white coats but in nylon shorts and T-shirts. We were distance runners: seven miles on weekdays, twelve miles on weekends. We pushed the pace until our legs cramped and our breath came in short gasps. We trained for marathons. Even outside of work, everything we did, we did to the maximum.

And it was that maximalist mind-set that resulted in the signature medical mistake of my life. One Sunday morning in Los Angeles, feeling fine, I stood up from a chair and nearly collapsed from excruciating back pain. The pain persisted for weeks, and the doctors I consulted had no ready explanation for it. But I was sure that medical science could pinpoint the cause of my pain. There had to be a fix somewhere in the universe of physicians and procedures.

I have written before about my back surgery, how I underwent the most aggressive operation, a spinal fusion, and its disastrous consequences: worsening pain and increased debility. But only when my wife and coauthor Pam and I began to think about this book, speaking in depth with patients about what guided their choices, reading studies in psychology and cognition, did I see how my mind as a patient had worked. In the early 1980s, there was already a school of clinical thought that most cases of back pain lacked a clear anatomical cause and that we can return to health by essentially doing nothing more than gradually moving about and waiting for the pain to pass.

But I lacked the patience to wait. I was headstrong, intolerant of the lack of an explanation for my misery. And I didn't believe that my body would heal itself. A naturalism bias was contrary to the beliefs of my childhood and the creed of my mentors.

The aggressive and unsuccessful surgery was a hard lesson in questioning my mind-set. It now seems self-evident, but mistakes are often necessary to bring insights. I learned to pay more attention to risk, to take time to consider side effects. Loss aversion can be a steadying force in making clinical choices. Pam took this cautious approach to medicine from the outset, and I moved closer to her thinking.

So when I reached my forties and found that my cholesterol level was 242, I had to decide whether to take a statin medication or forgo it. My father's tragic death impelled me to confront the reality that elevated lipids plagued our family; our genetics were inescapable. Not only had he died from a heart attack at an early age, but his two brothers, my uncles, also had coronary artery disease.

But the failed spinal surgery had made me risk-averse, particularly to anything that might affect my muscles, after years of suffering back pain. And as it happened, like Susan Powell, I had an acquaintance who had taken a statin medication and developed severe muscle inflammation. He was a doctor at our hospital, and one day in the parking lot, I saw him hobble away from his car. I thought he might have developed a degenerative neurological disorder, but he told me that he had taken a statin medication for an elevated cholesterol. Although many months had passed since he had stopped the drug, his muscle pain still had not subsided. I knew this was an anecdote, an "*n* of 1," but it made a deep impression on me. Availability, dramatic stories of benefit and of harm, affect us all, patient and physician alike.

So when my internist wanted to prescribe a statin, I declined at first. I had pivoted 180 degrees from my prior orientation. I would take a natural approach. Of course, you don't recalibrate your mindset completely. I was still a maximalist—I zealously adhered to a very strict diet, lost twelve pounds, exercised even more intensively. Six months later, my cholesterol had fallen four points to 238.

Although I was about a decade younger than my father was when he died, I felt that I had entered the phase of life where, like all the men in my family, I was marked for heart disease. I had to do something more.

My primary care physician suggested I begin on a standard dose of a statin, but I negotiated with him. "Let's begin at half dose," I said. I was aware that side effects were often dependent on dose. Although still committed to a natural approach, still strict about diet and exercise, I was forced to compromise. You can always increase the dose, I told myself. I would begin with a half step.

In six weeks, my total cholesterol was 160, and my "good" cholesterol, or HDL, was above 60. My muscles were not affected, then or in the ensuing years.

I was gratified, and not only because of the better numbers; I had understood my preferences and followed a deliberative process, reflecting on my thinking and acting in a way that makes sense to me.

[Pam's Narrative]

My father, an engineer, enthusiastically applied scientific principles to child rearing. When I, the first child, was born, he studied Dr. Truby King's method and decided that I would be fed on schedule, every four hours. He gave my mother a chart, carefully reviewing the plan before he left for work. After I screamed nonstop for two days, my mother, an artist and freethinker, took matters into her own hands: She fed me whenever she thought I was hungry. When my father asked how she could deviate from expert advice, my mother had a ready answer: "Doctors don't know everything."

My mother was ahead of her time with regard to a healthy diet. My friends had marshmallow cereal, Wonder bread sandwiches, and Twinkies. Not in our house. We had peanut butter and honey on whole-wheat bread with carrot sticks. In the 1950s, whole-wheat bread had not reached its current culinary heights; ours tasted like a mix of cardboard and sawdust. Fruit for dessert, no cookies. Milk with meals, no soda.

My father was an early riser and an avid exerciser. When the Royal Canadian Air Force exercise program was published in 1961, he became a fan and encouraged my sisters and me to follow the program with him, carefully measuring our progress. Although we didn't have much money, he decided that we should all learn to ski. So nearly every weekend, we all piled into our old station wagon and drove from New Jersey to Vermont, where we rented a large, dilapidated house along with several other families. All the children stayed together in a large, drafty dormitory in the attic. Undeterred by cold, ice, and wind, we rode the rope tows and skied all day until dusk.

When my youngest sister was five years old, she developed abdominal pain and fever. My mother brought her to the pediatrician who was covering the practice of our regular doctor. "It's nothing, just a virus," he reassured her.

It seemed that he was right, because the symptoms improved after a day or two. But the next week, my family was awakened late at night by my sister's shrieks. The abdominal pain was back, but much worse, and now she had a dangerously high fever. My mother plunged her into an ice bath and called the pediatrician. "Get her to the emergency room right now!" he said.

My sister's appendix had ruptured and bacteria had spread throughout her abdomen—peritonitis. In retrospect, her initial symptoms the week before had been the early signs of appendicitis. I vividly recall visiting my sister in the hospital, hiding in the corner as the nurse entered the room carrying a metal tray containing two syringes topped with gigantic needles. I fled the room in horror before my sister received these painful antibiotic injections into her buttocks and thighs; they were given every two hours. The lesson was clear: Doctors were not always right.

My father was fascinated by science and medicine and wished that he could have become a doctor. When I was young, he encouraged me to be a nurse. As more opportunities opened for women, I decided I would become a doctor. I attended what was then Radcliffe College at Harvard University and immersed myself in science. I had inherited my father's facility with numbers and was first drawn to the quantitative sciences: advanced mathematics, physics, biophysical chemistry. I enjoyed working with formulas that gave clear and precise answers. But I was also drawn to biology with its inherent variability, where the correct answer could not always be predicted, where normal was not a number but a range, a continuum without clear cutoffs.

My first personal encounter with illness occurred when I was a senior in college. I woke one morning with an intense and painful urge to urinate. When I looked down at the toilet bowl, it was red with blood. Terrified, I ran to the student health service, where an experienced nurse-practitioner reassured me that I was not dying. "It's nothing serious," she said, "just a bladder infection, easily treated with antibiotics." She gave me a prescription for a sulfa drug and told me to call her if I had any problems.

I picked up the medication from a local pharmacy. Enclosed with the medication bottle was a package insert with detailed information about the antibiotic, including a very long list of possible side effects. I read carefully through this information: severe total body rash, liver failure, even death. I was paralyzed. Should I really take this dangerous drug? Did this nurse-practitioner actually know what she was doing? But my symptoms were too much to bear, so with trepidation I put a pill in my mouth and swallowed it down, fully convinced that I would develop some terrible side effect. I didn't, and within a day my symptoms were gone. Despite this therapeutic success, I remained, like my mother, a doubter. But being a doubter did not stop me from becoming a doctor.

As a student at Harvard Medical School, I found that my most inspiring teachers were endocrinologists. They seemed to know all of medicine, alert to subtleties in the individual patient's history and physical exam that could easily be overlooked. Snoring, excessive sweating, and a change in shoe size were all caused by an excess of growth hormone from the pituitary gland. A tan that did not fade hid a failing adrenal gland. A tremor of the hands and discomfort in the eyes indicated an excess of thyroid hormone. One hormone regulated another via elegant feedback loops that kept the body in balance.

After completing my training in endocrinology and metabolism, I became interested in the issue of hormone replacement for menopausal women. In the 1980s and early 1990s, treatment with estrogen, usually in combination with another hormone called progestin, had become standard practice, not only to ameliorate menopausal symptoms of hot flashes, but also to protect women from osteoporosis and most important to prevent heart disease, stroke, and dementia. As a doubter, I remained skeptical that these hormones could prevent so many of the consequences of aging. And being risk-averse, I was concerned about the downsides of estrogen, especially the risk of breast cancer.

In researching this topic for lectures to physicians and lay audiences, I was bothered by the fact that the Framingham Heart Study, the largest and one of the best long-term epidemiological surveys, didn't show a clear benefit of estrogen on the heart. It became difficult for me to recommend estrogen treatment to all my patients, and I felt the decision to prescribe it needed to be individualized. In 2002, the Women's Health Initiative found through a controlled trial that hormone replacement therapy (HRT) for menopausal women did not prevent heart disease; in fact, it appeared to increase the risk of heart attack. Similarly, HRT did not prevent Alzheimer's disease or other forms of dementia. Finally, the risk of breast cancer was increased with hormonal treatment. The issue of hormone therapy for menopause is still much debated.

When it comes to my own health, I am a minimalist, and I don't like to take medicines or supplements unless absolutely necessary. I worry about side effects from medications and from diagnostic and therapeutic procedures for myself and for my patients.

Nearly ten years ago in the winter, I began to lose weight. At first I was delighted, attributing it to my increased hours of tennis and skiing. But the weight loss persisted over several months despite eating more and cutting back on exercise. And I noticed that my endurance was less than usual. I tried to ignore or explain away my symptoms.

But finally, when I became so short of breath during a tennis match that I had to stop playing and sit down on the court, I realized that something was really wrong. The diagnosis turned out to be Graves' disease, an overactive thyroid gland. Although it was not a big surprise because many of the women in my family have thyroid disease, the diagnosis was not immediately obvious to me or to my physician husband, Jerry. Once the diagnosis was made, I had to face the reality that therapy was unavoidable. I had treated many patients with Graves' disease in my endocrinology practice, and I was well versed in the benefits and risks of each treatment approach. In addition, I had the benefit of many patient stories to call upon in making the decision that was right for me.

Several years later, I was injured in a ski accident. While waiting for my children at the bottom of a hill, a young man came bombing out of the trees, smashed into me, and knocked me over. Fortunately no bones were broken, but my ankle was twisted, painful, and swollen. For months I was sidelined from playing tennis, and even walking was uncomfortable. Restless from lack of exercise, I went to the hospital on a Sunday to clean out my office. I did a deep knee bend to pick up a large pile of books and heard a loud pop in my knee. The joint immediately swelled to the size of a grapefruit and was exquisitely painful. I tried ice and a knee brace, but the pain and swelling persisted. Finally, after a week of hobbling around, I made an appointment with an orthopedic surgeon. He examined me, pointed out my flat feet that put me at risk for knee injury, and recommended an MRI scan, which was booked for one week later. On the day I was to have the scan, I saw one of my patients who has a deep doubter mind-set. She saw my limp, and when she heard that I was scheduled for an MRI, she looked at me and said, "But Doctor, you once told me that it can take weeks for a knee injury to heal. Why are you having an MRI so soon?" I decided to postpone the scan. Sure enough, about ten days later the knee was fine, and I was soon back to full activity. I never did get that MRI scan.

Over time, much of my clinical practice has focused on thyroid disease and thyroid cancer. I now serve as medical director of our hospital's thyroid nodule clinic, where patients with growths in the thyroid gland come for evaluation and biopsy. Thyroid cancers are often found incidentally on examination or on imaging done for other reasons. Most of these thyroid cancers are small, slow growing, and easily cured. My minimalist mind-set fits well with a tempered approach appropriate to treating this kind of tumor. But some thyroid cancers are extremely aggressive and require equally aggressive treatment. Caring for such patients, I deliberately shift my mind-set and become a maximalist.

My parents, now in their eighties, continue to be active and in generally good health. My father enjoys discussing new developments in science and medicine with me. My mother still tells me what to eat, pointing out that salmon and blueberries are healthy and that I should be sure to get enough calcium. When I point out that I am a doctor, her response is, "Well, doctors don't know everything." And of course, she is correct.

[Joint Conclusion]

Despite working in medicine as physicians for more than thirty years, we were surprised to realize that we had had only a hazy understanding of our own mind-sets. Revisiting our family history, our prior medical history, and our social history opened our eyes to the origin and nature of our preferences about our own health. We were struck by similarities to the patients we'd spoken to. Like Michelle Byrd, one of us was a believer in maximizing treatment and had a strong technology orientation; the other, like Susan Powell, was a doubter, risk-averse, and in favor of minimal treatment.

In our role as doctors, our aim is to help our patients understand what makes sense for them, what treatments are right given their individual values and goals. We are especially mindful not to impose our preferences about our own health on our patients.

Three

—————

But Is It Best for Me?

Patrick Baptiste, a thirty-six-year-old personal trainer at a popular health club in Houston, Texas, typically bench-pressed 310 to 320 pounds. Standing just shy of six feet three inches, with broad shoulders and a neatly trimmed goatee, Patrick had a warm and relaxed manner that made him one of the favorite instructors among patrons of the gym. One day shortly before Thanksgiving, when he positioned himself squarely on the bench to show a new member how to press properly, the weight seemed unusually heavy. Over the ensuing months, his strength seemed to decline, until he strained to press 225 pounds. Patrick had been eating more than usual to boost his strength and was surprised when he got on the scale and saw that he had lost seven pounds. He looked at himself in the mirror and noticed that the prominent curves of his biceps seemed a little flatter. Even more perplexing were several episodes of rapid heartbeat and trembling in his hands. These episodes occurred not only after he worked out at the gym, but once when he was driving to visit his family on a day off and another time when he was stretched out on his couch watching football. Patrick often felt on edge and several times was impatient with clients at the gym. Finally, when he realized that it took effort even to walk up a flight of stairs, he went to see his primary care doctor.

Patrick's physician had cared for him for several years and noted that his pulse, normally in the low 60s typical for an athlete, was now 90. As the doctor examined him, he stopped at his neck. "You have a muscular neck," the doctor said, "so I'm not sure, but your thyroid gland seems a little enlarged. That might explain what's going on here." The physician performed blood tests and called Patrick the next day to say that his thyroid hormone levels were too high. "I'm going to send you to an endocrinologist who specializes in thyroid conditions," the doctor said. "In the meantime, this medication will help with some of your symptoms, and you should start to feel better." He prescribed a medication called a "beta-blocker" to alleviate the tremor and slow the rapid heartbeat. "Before you see the specialist, we'll get a scan of your thyroid. He'll review the results and decide on the best therapy."

The specialist's office was not far from Patrick's health club. After a short wait, he was ushered into an exam room. The doctor asked Patrick how he was feeling and then handed him a glass of water. He asked Patrick to sip and swallow several times as he stared intently at the front of Patrick's neck. He then stood behind Patrick, placed his fingers around both sides of his neck, and again asked him to swallow. Taking his stethoscope from his pocket, he listened over Patrick's neck. Finally, the doctor took out what looked like a metal ruler and measured the distance from the corner to the front of Patrick's eyes. He put down the instrument and went back to his desk.

"You have Graves' disease, a form of hyperthyroidism, an overactive thyroid gland." The doctor swiveled his computer screen so that

Patrick could see it. "Here, take a look at this scan of your thyroid," the doctor said. The image looked like a huge stippled butterfly. "The best treatment for this condition is radioactive iodine. You swallow a radioactive pill, and it destroys the gland. Problem solved. You get it over with." The doctor paused. "After that you'll just need a daily thyroid pill. No big deal."

But, Patrick told us, for him it was a "big deal."

He asked the endocrinologist what alternatives there might be to radioactive iodine. "There are other options, but they're not as good. This is clearly the best treatment."

But Patrick persisted. "What are the other options?"

"There are medications that prevent the thyroid gland from making too much hormone," the doctor said. "But these drugs sometimes have terrible side effects, damaging your liver or knocking down the white blood cell count so you could be open to life-threatening infections." The doctor paused for a few moments, seeming to let that information sink in. "Or you could have surgery to remove the gland. But that also has real risks, with anesthesia, bleeding, and the possibility of damaging the other glands in the neck, the parathyroid glands, or even injuring the nerves to your vocal cords. This is really the best option."

Patrick felt unsettled by the doctor's words. "I don't trust this idea of one-size-fits-all when it comes to medical problems," he told us. His skepticism was the paradoxical gift of a previous illness, diabetes, diagnosed in his teens. Patrick was the oldest of five children, all born after his family had emigrated from Haiti and settled near relatives in Houston. As a teenager, already at six feet two inches, he weighed 260 pounds, and was a defensive lineman on the high school varsity football team. His mother, father, and grandparents all had diabetes. At age nineteen, when Patrick developed periods of intense thirst and frequent urination, classic signs of diabetes, his mother used one of her own test strips and found sugar in his urine. For several years he had taken oral medication and, at times, insulin injections to control his blood sugar.

Initially, Patrick said, his adherence to his prescribed diabetes therapy might well be described as "pretty poor." Like many of his age, he often skipped his medication, so that his blood sugar swung widely. "My diet was terrible, chips and soda, because I wanted to be normal, like all the other kids," he said. His doctors and his mother warned Patrick about the kidney failure and blindness that can result from uncontrolled diabetes, but these warnings had no effect on him. "It was hard to really imagine that you might get those kinds of complications," he recalled. "They seemed far off, irrelevant. But when the doctors told me that I could become impotent, that got my attention." Diabetics are vulnerable to nerve damage because the small blood vessels that feed the nerves can become diseased; if the nerves in the penis suffer this complication of the disorder, impotence results. "Finally, I heard something that was really important to me. It motivated me to take my diabetes seriously, and I began to take care of myself and follow the doctor's advice."

Patrick lost weight, and on a carefully controlled diet and a regular regimen of exercise, his blood sugar returned to normal. Now he took only one pill a day to keep his diabetes in check and didn't need insulin. Patrick told us that when he first developed his symptoms of hyperthyroidism, he thought it might be due to his diabetes, that his sugar was out of control. But it wasn't.

Because his insurance coverage had changed a few times over the years, Patrick had seen several diabetes specialists, and he'd discovered that they didn't all agree on what was best for him, which oral medications to take, whether or not he should also be on insulin, and even how tightly he should regulate his blood sugar. "I know from my own work as a trainer that you need to individualize exercise regimens, because different bodies advance at different speeds." Whenever Patrick worked with a client at the gym, he tried to define the person's goals, desired weight, and level of fitness, and then they worked together, regularly assessing whether they were on the right track or needed to rethink their approach. He couldn't imagine telling a client that there was one "best" path to fitness.

Although Patrick had no prior knowledge of Graves' disease or the options for treatment, he felt he was being told—too quickly and too definitively—that there was one "best" approach. As it happens, clinical research supports Patrick's thinking. A group of endocrinologists at the Karolinska University Hospital in Stockholm, Sweden, conducted a study to assess the benefits and risks of the three common treatments for Graves' disease. They randomly assigned 179 patients to take antithyroid medication, undergo surgery on their thyroid gland, or receive radioactive iodine; the follow-up time was at least four years. The study showed that all three treatments were equally effective in controlling the disorder. Importantly, 90 percent of the patients were satisfied with their treatment—no matter which treatment they'd had—and would recommend it to a friend.

What Patrick experienced with his endocrinologist reflects a common and understandable phenomenon: The doctor projects his or her own preferences onto the patient. This has been documented in studies of a wide variety of conditions ranging from asthma to autoimmune arthritis of the spine, from prostate cancer to esophageal disease. Here, the endocrinologist truly believed that radioiodine therapy was best. His reasons for preferring this treatment were that it was simple—one radioiodine pill—and definitive—"problem solved." But not every endocrinologist shares this view. An international survey of thyroid specialists showed that about two-thirds of American endocrinologists favored radioiodine for treatment of Graves' disease, but only 22 percent of European and 11 percent of Japanese specialists did. Outside the United States, endocrinologists favored antithyroid drugs. Endocrinologists around the world have access to the same data from clinical studies and are schooled in the risks and benefits of each treatment. Yet the default option, presented as what is "best" for the patient, is strikingly different in these three regions. Part of the reason for this difference is likely cultural. The Japanese experience with nuclear weapons at Hiroshima and Nagasaki undoubtedly colors their views on radiation exposure. The 2011 earthquake and tsunami that damaged the nuclear reactors in Japan will likely amplify this. Western Europe is also leery of radiation, and this attitude was later reinforced by the accident at the Chernobyl nuclear plant.

The search for the "best choice" takes us to an eighteenth-century Dutch mathematician named Daniel Bernoulli. At the time, Holland was a hub of world commerce, and its traders were making decisions about buying and selling everything from Asian spices to Caribbean sugarcane. Bernoulli was born in the city of Groningen in 1700. His father, a mathematician, encouraged him to study business to assure himself a good income. At first, Bernoulli refused. Later, he agreed to study both business and medicine, but only under the condition that his father instruct him privately in mathematics. He ultimately became a professor of medicine, metaphysics, and natural philosophy at the University of Basel in Switzerland. His seminal work in fluid mechanics helps explain how birds fly and was crucial to the development of airplanes. In 1738, he turned his attention to probability theory and devised a formula that he believed would calculate the wisdom of any decision where the outcome was uncertain and the choice involved risk. He proposed that by multiplying the probability or chance of an outcome by the utility of that outcome, meaning how much we value it, we obtain a number, the "expected utility." The highest number, the greatest "expected utility," indicates the most rational choice.

[(probability of outcome) × (utility of outcome) = expected utility]

Bernoulli was thinking mostly about choices that involved goods and money, and his formula for "rational" decision making has been widely applied in economics. Over the last few decades, however, "expected utility" theory has moved beyond economics and into clinical medicine. Researchers have proposed that doctors should advise a patient like Patrick Baptiste of his best option by using Bernoulli's calculations. First, the physician would tell Patrick the probability of a clinical outcome and then ask him to place a numerical value or "utility" on his health state if that outcome occurred. Multiplying the chance that a particular outcome might occur by the numerical value Patrick placed on living with that outcome yields a number; the highest number indicates his most rational or "best" choice.

This formula has great appeal, as it pinpoints two key components we all should consider when choosing among different options: what is likely to happen and how our life would be affected if it did happen. All of us want to live the longest life with the highest quality. In the case of Graves' disease, all three options—radioiodine, surgery, medication—can yield the desired positive outcome, control of hyperthyroidism. But there are differences in potential negative outcomes and side effects, as well as in quality of life in the future.

Let's first imagine that the endocrinologist advising Patrick used Bernoulli's equation. As all the treatments can be effective in controlling hyperthyroidism, the probability of this outcome is equivalent for all three therapies. What differs are the potential side effects. Patrick's physician views the side effects of antithyroid medication and surgery as much more serious than those of radioactive iodine. So he would assign these treatments a lower "utility" or value, and he would logically arrive at treatment with radioactive iodine as the best option. He framed his discussion with Patrick in these terms.

But Patrick would solve the same equation quite differently. He cringed when the endocrinologist said that it was "no big deal" to destroy his thyroid gland with radioactive iodine so that he would have to take a thyroid hormone pill every day for the rest of his life. "I don't like having to take medication every day for my diabetes. And I didn't want to commit myself to taking another pill every day—to have another chronic condition." He explained that "when I watched my diet, exercised, and controlled my weight, I was able to come off insulin injections. But if you destroy the thyroid gland, this is permanent—I have no opportunity to get off that thyroid pill."

Patrick views the need to take thyroid medication permanently in strongly negative terms. So for him, radioactive iodine and surgery have much less "utility" than antithyroid medication and would not be valued as "best" for him.

Of course, another patient might solve this equation differently.

Anna Gonzales, a forty-two-year-old journalist with three teenage children and a hectic schedule, also developed Graves' disease. When her endocrinologist suggested treatment with radioactive iodine, she readily agreed. "I want this taken care of quickly," she explained. When we asked her if she was bothered by the idea of taking a pill every day, she replied, "Well, I already take a birth control pill. This is not a problem for me."

Lily Chan, a twenty-seven-year-old social worker, chose surgery for treatment of her Graves' disease. "I'm really afraid of radioactive iodine," she told us. "No one can guarantee 100 percent that I won't have some kind of side effect that is not known about now, maybe even cancer."

But Patrick had no fear of radiation and no particular bias against surgery. "I simply don't want to be forced to take another pill every day for the rest of my life," he told us.

In the field of decision analysis, the utility or value that a person assigns to a particular outcome is termed his "preference." Researchers have found that patients often construct their preferences on the spot when the doctor gives a diagnosis and recommends a treatment. Such patients are something of a "blank slate" upon which the doctor can "write" his or her own preference. In this setting, the patient is especially susceptible to how the physician frames the pros and cons of the treatment.

The endocrinologist who advised Patrick framed his remarks in a way that clearly reflected his own bias by emphasizing the side effects of treatments other than radioactive iodine. He presented radioactive iodine as the standard or "default" option. Research in behavioral psychology shows that most people will accept the default option; they assume that what is routinely recommended is "best." It takes effort for a non-expert to decline the default option and seek an alternative. But that's exactly what Patrick did. Because of his prior experiences with diabetes, he'd developed certain views about health. He wasn't a "blank slate," and he didn't construct his preferences on the spot. For him, past was prologue.

We should then ask why Patrick's endocrinologist had such a strong bias for radioactive iodine and framed his advice as he did. Perhaps he'd had bad experiences with antithyroid medications, where a patient had suffered a sharp drop in white blood cell count and developed a serious infection; or perhaps one of his patients had suffered serious complications from thyroid surgery. If so, this would reflect an "availability" bias: a dramatic past case readily recalled that colored the doctor's thinking. But it simply may be that the endocrinologist was conforming to the cultural preference of his colleagues in the United States and that if he had been practicing in Europe or Japan, he would have conformed to the prevailing biases in those regions.

Patrick Baptiste had accepted and adapted to one chronic condition, diabetes. He felt that adding a second chronic condition, permanent hypothyroidism that required daily treatment, would deeply disturb his life. Such strongly held personal views are at times difficult for others to fathom. The endocrinologist who evaluated Patrick could not understand why adding one more pill could be a "big deal." Indeed, as physicians, we often prescribe medication with the assumption that it is "no big deal." And we assume that the patient will feel the same. However, a study of common medical conditions—including osteoarthritis of the hip and knee, benign enlargement of the prostate gland, or a ruptured disk—found significant differences in how patients and physicians weighed the goals and consequences of available treatments, including the burden of taking daily medication. Patients should be aware that doctors and other experts may frame information in a way that reflects their own preferences. As physicians, we've both found ourselves at times too quickly telling our patients which treatments we prefer rather than working with them to understand their own thinking. Of course, patients may want, and often ask, what their physicians think is best. But that should occur after information is presented in a neutral way.

This divide between doctors' and patients' preferences has been studied in depth in treatment of another problem, atrial fibrillation, the condition that affected Dave Simon. This abnormal cardiac rhythm is very common: About 1 percent of Americans in their fifties suffer from it, and 5 to 10 percent of those who are seventy or older do. Based on data from the Framingham Heart Study, it is estimated that over the course of a lifetime, atrial fibrillation or a related rhythm called atrial flutter will occur in about 25 percent of the population. It can be the first sign of hyperthyroidism, especially in the elderly.

Atrial fibrillation occurs when the upper part of the heart called the atrium contracts abnormally, so that the heart beats in a disorganized and irregular way. Blood can pool in the heart, and clots can form. These clots can then be pumped out to the body and result in a stroke. Patients with atrial fibrillation are often treated with "blood-thinning" medications called anticoagulants, like warfarin or aspirin, that help prevent clots from forming. But these treatments can cause profuse bleeding. Such hemorrhaging is most common in the gastrointestinal tract but can be particularly devastating when it occurs in the brain. So the patient with atrial fibrillation must choose whether to take medication that may prevent a stroke from a clot but can cause serious bleeding.

Researchers at Dalhousie University in Nova Scotia interviewed sixty physicians who were treating patients with atrial fibrillation. They also interviewed a similar number of patients who did not have atrial fibrillation but were at high risk for developing this condition. Each doctor and each patient was asked to consider treatment options for a theoretical group of one hundred patients who had atrial fibrillation: Options included no therapy, aspirin, or warfarin. Both the doctors and the patients were presented the same numerical information about the chances of stroke and bleeding for each option and then were asked if the treatment was justified. The patients placed significantly more value or "utility" on avoiding stroke, while the physicians placed more value on avoiding bleeding. Although there was no information about why the doctors valued the risks and benefits of the treatment differently from the patients, the researchers concluded, "The views of the individual patient should be considered when decisions are being made about treatment for people with atrial fibrillation."

Researchers at the Ottawa Hospital in Canada similarly studied nearly two hundred patients from sixty to eighty years old who didn't have atrial fibrillation but were likely to develop the condition in the future. These patients were asked to imagine that they themselves had atrial fibrillation and to consider if they would take anticoagulants for it. One group received information using qualitative language, where risk of stroke or bleeding was designated as either "low" or "moderate." The other group received detailed quantitative data on stroke and bleeding risks, carefully framed in both positive and negative ways—for example, "3 out of 100 chance of stroke, meaning 97 out of 100 chance of *not* having a stroke with treatment."

In this study, patients given the most detailed information chose what researchers termed "the extremes" of treatment; more participants chose either the potent anticoagulant warfarin or no treatment at all rather than the middle-of-the-road option, aspirin. Giving more exact and understandable clinical information brought out greater individual differences in patients' preferences.

Dave Simon, the avid tennis player with atrial fibrillation whom you met at the beginning of this book, was poised to make a serious treatment decision—caught between two images of the future, a stroke or severe hemorrhage. To complicate matters, a brand-new medication had just become available. This new blood thinner required less monitoring than warfarin, and studies showed a somewhat smaller risk of bleeding. But slightly more people had heart attacks while on this new drug, for unclear reasons. Dave's cardiologist offered him the standard treatment options as well as this new medication. She showed Dave the number needed to treat with each drug, how many people needed to receive the medication to prevent one stroke from occurring. The doctor also informed Dave of what is termed "the number needed to harm," meaning how many people typically must receive the drug for one person to have a serious side effect, in this case bleeding into the gastrointestinal tract or brain.

Dave went through a deliberate process, not only examining these numbers, but also considering his mind-set. Dave had a doubter approach to treatments. He was afraid to take any of these medications, but he realized he was more terrified of having a stroke. After several sleepless nights, he made his decision. "I decided to stick with the traditional blood thinner," he told us. "I'm not an early adopter. I remembered what happened a few years ago with Vioxx, how excited everyone was about it and how doctors said it was so much better than aspirin and other drugs. Then they found out that it caused heart attacks, too. I prefer to take a medication with a longer track record." Someone else with a believer orientation might eagerly greet the news of a new anticoagulant and request to be switched to it, even if he was doing well on his current therapy.

A team of researchers studying therapy of high blood pressure made a similar observation about the wide variety of patient preferences. In this study, researchers presented a series of scenarios about hypertension therapy to both physicians and patients. Physicians and patients then were asked to determine at what point the benefits of therapy outweighed the risk of side effects, cost, and inconvenience. The researchers found that given the same information, patients were generally less likely than doctors to accept treatment for high blood pressure. The patients tended to be more risk-averse, weighing the side effects of the medications more heavily than their doctors did.

In this study, one-third of the patients interviewed decided against drug therapy for high blood pressure when presented with a scenario that would qualify them for treatment based on expert opinion. Like Alex Miller, these patients didn't want the therapy recommended by their doctors. But the researchers also found that a significant subgroup of patients (15 to 20 percent) wanted treatment that had no proven benefit and was not recommended. We would term these patients maximalists—like Michelle Byrd. These people often feel that they're "ahead of the curve" in protecting their health, even though scientific data do not yet support their view.

Patients should be aware that there can be differing views among specialists about who should be treated for various conditions. For example, expert committees in Europe and the United States crafted different guidelines about when to treat high blood pressure. The group of American experts believed that the benefits outweighed the risks from treatment for mild elevation of blood pressure and wrote guidelines that advise medication for patients like Alex Miller. But in Europe, an expert committee with access to the same scientific data formulated different guidelines that don't advise treatment for mild elevation of blood pressure. In Europe, Alex and others like him would not be encouraged to take medication. Different groups of experts can disagree significantly about what is "best practice."

Dr. Rodney Hayward, a widely respected researcher on health care at the University of Michigan, recently wrote in the *New England Journal of Medicine* that "the assessment of whether the benefit is great enough to warrant the risk of harm—i.e., the decision of where the threshold for intervention should lie—is necessarily a value judgment."

Why is it subjective, a value judgment, rather than a matter of a clear black-and-white answer? Because, Hayward continues, for many treatments there exists a substantial "gray area of indeterminate net benefit."

Hayward mentions cholesterol levels as one example of such a gray area. We examined the "net benefit" of treatment in Susan Powell's deliberation about taking a statin medication. "Net benefit" means the potential gains from the treatment minus the downsides. After seeing all the data, particularly the "number needed to treat," she didn't believe the net benefit was worth it, given the risks statins entail. In effect, Susan set a different cutoff for herself from the one some experts would apply, not because she was "health illiterate" or "irrational," but because she has a different subjective assessment from that of the experts who wrote the recommendations. We agree strongly with Hayward that within the substantial gray area of indeterminate net benefit, "physicians should defer to an individual patient's preferences in choosing whether or not to intervene."

How do recommendations for "best practice" come about? Committees of specialists are convened to draw up guidelines that aim to identify "best practice" for a certain medical condition. The principle is that guidelines should be drawn from the "best" evidence and crafted by the "best" scientific experts in the field. These guidelines are a key component of so-called evidence-based medicine, the idea that clinical practice should be based solely on the results of scientific studies. The recommendations are presented not only to physicians, but directly to patients, in informational brochures, on the Internet, and in the media. Guidelines therefore have become one of the most powerful forces on patient decisions, since the very language used to describe their content is "best" practice. Advocates of guidelines assert that both doctors and patients should accept their recommendations as the default option. Some physicians and health policy planners conclude that patients who deviate from expert recommendations aren't adequately informed or are "irrational."

Doctors and patients certainly should consult guidelines since they provide considerable background information about disorders and treatment options. But, it's important to recognize that guidelines aren't strictly "scientific." They incorporate biases and subjective judgments. Experts select which clinical studies to use and which to discard when they formulate their recommendations. Further, all studies have limitations. They provide results from statistical averages of selected groups of study subjects. These averages may not be applicable to a particular patient. Even the most rigorous, inclusive studies cannot address all the variables of age, gender, genetics, lifestyle, diet, and concurrent medical conditions that make us individuals and often influence how effective a particular treatment will be or what sorts of side effects we might experience. Many studies exclude the elderly or those who have coexisting common medical problems. When making their final recommendations about the need for treatment, experts also apply their subjective judgment about how much risk is worth taking in order to obtain a certain benefit. Concerns have also been raised by the Institute of Medicine about potential conflicts of interest, since some experts who write guidelines are consultants to drug and device companies or private insurers. Finally, guideline committees have an imperative for consensus and present their recommendations with one voice. As a result, their conclusions usually fail to mention dissenting opinions that may have arisen among committee members.

It's also important for patients to realize that guidelines aren't engraved in stone; they can change quickly. A survey of one hundred recommendations from expert committees found that within a year 14 percent were reversed, within two years 23 percent were changed, and fully half were overturned at five and a half years. The American College of Physicians, representing internists in the United States, stated in 2010 that all of its guidelines, if not rewritten, should be automatically suspended after five years. This isn't only because new and better data become available, but also because the composition of expert committees may change, and with this change, subjective judgments of "utility" or value may shift. Consider the guidelines that recommended the use of estrogen in virtually all postmenopausal women to prevent heart disease and dementia. These guidelines were overturned by new information from the Women's Health Initiative trial. Yet some experts remain critical of this study and still endorse parts of the earlier guidelines, believing that for some women the "value" of hormone replacement may be enough to risk the downsides.

Clearly, more than assessments of scientific evidence, more than extracting numbers from clinical research, goes into guidelines and their recommendations. The conclusions drawn about what is "best" necessarily incorporate the second part of the Bernoulli formula, the "value" or impact of a treatment on quality of life. For every individual, this impact is always subjective and cannot be distilled from objective data.

We believe that all patients should be fully informed about their condition and then asked about their preferences. Such "informed patient preference" is placed by the Institute of Medicine of the National Academy of Sciences at the pinnacle of "quality care." To be truly informed, patients should be aware of the gray zones in medicine. They must keep in mind that guidelines are not purely scientific and have a significant subjective component.

In 2010, researchers at the University of Michigan published the results of one of the first national surveys of medical decisions. The researchers contacted at random by telephone 3,100 adults age forty and older. Participants were asked a series of questions about common medical conditions they might have discussed with their doctors. A disturbing finding was that only half the patients stated they had been asked their preferences about starting medications for elevated blood pressure or a high cholesterol level. Although guidelines usually have fine print at the bottom asserting that the recommendations need to be molded to the preferences, values, and goals of the individual patient, we believe that this statement should be in large print, because patient preference is often not sought.

There is a creeping paternalism on the part of health care policy makers and insurance companies to standardize care based on guidelines. To be sure, standardization is appropriate, even essential, in some areas of medicine, like safety measures and emergency care. But where patient preferences are involved, standardization is misconceived. Yet, there are powerful incentives, often financial, to reward doctors when their patients receive treatment according to guidelines and penalize them when their patients deviate from the recommendations. Report cards that rate physicians according to compliance with guidelines are issued by insurers and often made public. We readily see how a physician might feel caught by these incentives and press patients to make choices that may not reflect either physician or patient preferences. As a patient, you want to know that your doctor is on your side, helping you to figure out an individual choice.

What if you and your physician don't agree about what is the "best" choice? In such settings, as Dr. Jacques Carter put it, physicians "negotiate" with their patient. But the ultimate choice is always the patient's, because it is the patient who either enjoys the benefit of a treatment or suffers its side effects, experiencing each within the context of his or her values and goals in life.

Patrick Baptiste had a different assessment from that of the endocrinologist about the risks and benefits of his treatment. He returned to his primary care doctor, who at his request referred him to another endocrinologist. "This doctor laid out all three options and gave me the pros and cons on each." The physician didn't immediately present one way as the best. "Instead, he asked me what I thought about each option."

The new doctor explained to Patrick that antithyroid medication could control the hyperthyroidism until the Graves' disease entered remission. But he also made it clear there was no guarantee that he would go into remission or that remission would be permanent.

"If I have at least a chance of going into remission and not have to add another pill and another chronic condition to my life, then to me, it's worth a try," Patrick said. "I realize that if it doesn't work, I may need to have radioactive iodine or surgery. But I'll deal with that if and when I get there."

Four

Regret

Lisa Norton walked quickly down the corridor to the classroom. A forty-two-year-old teacher of English as a second language in South Florida, she made it a point of pride never to be late for her students. As she neared the door, she was stopped by a knifelike pain in her foot. Lisa took a deep breath, composed her face, and entered the classroom, trying to hide any sign of discomfort.

That was eight months ago. At the time, an orthopedic surgeon had examined her foot, taken an X-ray, and told her that there was a bone spur at the first metatarsal joint, as well as a ganglion cyst and arthritis. "It needs surgery," the doctor said. "There is extensive degeneration there." He explained that in addition to removing the bone spur and cyst, he would place two small titanium screws and fuse the adjacent bones. The fusion would prevent the joint from moving, since any friction in such an arthritic joint would cause pain.

Lisa, a slim, athletic woman, had been a distance runner in college. She knew many runners who'd had joint pain and improved after receiving cortisone shots. Lisa asked the surgeon if she could try such a steroid injection.

"It won't work," the doctor said flatly.

But, Lisa told us, she had pressed him to give the shot, and it had worked. "I walked for eight months without any discomfort at all after the cortisone injection." But then the pain returned.

Lisa had strong ideas about treatment. At the age of twenty-four, at the peak of her performance as a runner, Lisa had developed severe fatigue, pain in her joints, and a rash on her cheeks. She was diagnosed with lupus, an autoimmune disease that can affect many of the body's tissues. She initially approached her therapy with a deep naturalism orientation. "I rested in bed for four months," Lisa said, "reading my wacky books, hoping that I would go into remission spontaneously, that my body would heal itself." But the symptoms did not improve, and "finally, I had so much pain and was so fatigued I could hardly move." She consulted with a rheumatologist, a specialist in autoimmune diseases, and was treated with high doses of prednisone and Imuran, drugs that inhibit the immune system.

Lisa regained her energy, and the pain in her joints and rash subsided. But, as often happens, she suffered side effects from these potent medications. Her face swelled, her appetite became voracious, and she couldn't sleep. She also worried that Imuran, which is toxic to blood cells, might make her more likely to develop cancer. "I kept trying to wean myself off the treatments," she told us, "only to have the lupus return and then have to go way back up on the doses of the drugs." Her rheumatologist "understood where I was coming from," acknowledging Lisa's concerns about the side effects of the potent medications and her desire to let the body heal itself. After several years, the autoimmune disease went into remission, and she no longer needed to take any medication. She hasn't required any further treatment for her lupus since then. During her illness, Lisa told us, "I learned to be an advocate for myself."

Lisa Norton's story gives insight into the experience of patients confronting serious conditions. When you feel good, it's difficult to imagine the choices and to forecast the decisions you will make when you are ill. When her lupus did not go away, as Lisa termed it, "through a natural path," with nutrition, meditation, relaxation techniques, and other approaches, her apparently fixed preferences became more flexible. New circumstances moved her to alter her mind-set. Yet she still retained her fundamental belief in a natural approach.

When the pain returned, Lisa rested at home with her foot elevated. Over the next few weeks, she tried icing the area and was fitted with new orthotics. But the pain didn't get any better. She returned to the surgeon.

"I'm not surprised," he said when Lisa told him about her condition. "You need surgery, I told you that before."

Lisa and her daughter had scheduled a trip to Europe in a few weeks' time. The trip had been planned for a long while, and she told the doctor that she didn't want an operation to interfere with it.

"You have pain from the bone spur, the ganglion cyst, and lots of arthritis in that joint," the doctor reiterated. "That's going to interfere with your trip. I can fix all of that, and in two weeks you'll be fine to travel."

"I'd rather have another cortisone shot," Lisa replied.

The doctor paused and then spoke deliberately, emphasizing each word. It sounded to Lisa as though he were speaking to a badly behaved child. "I will give you the shot. But this is not a cure. Let's get you on the schedule for surgery." Lisa agreed.

The trip to Europe was everything that Lisa and her daughter had hoped for. They both loved art, and they spent days lingering in the museums in Paris. Despite the many hours Lisa spent on her feet, she didn't feel any discomfort—the shot again had worked. But her surgery was already scheduled. So when she returned, she went to the hospital for her preoperative evaluation.

In the examination room, Lisa almost dozed off waiting to meet with the nurse who would clear her for surgery. Her jet lag still hadn't worn off. The nurse greeted Lisa with a warm smile and went over a checklist, reviewing Lisa's past medical history, asking about any allergies or reactions to medication. She noted the normal recent electrocardiogram and chest X-ray, which showed that Lisa was healthy enough to undergo surgery.

"You know," Lisa said, "my foot feels fine now. I wonder if I really have to have such an extensive surgery?"

The nurse glanced up from the paperwork and gave Lisa a quizzical look. "You really should discuss that with your doctor," she said. "But in any event, since you're here, let's get your pre-op blood tests done." The nurse handed Lisa a sheet with a series of tests marked off and told her how to find the phlebotomist who would draw her blood.

The next day at school, Lisa confirmed with the principal that her class would be covered by a substitute teacher for at least two weeks after the operation.

"You know, my foot feels good, even though I walked all over Paris," Lisa told her. "I wonder if I really need this kind of operation?"

The principal raised an eyebrow. "You should talk to your doctor," she suggested.

When we spoke with Lisa, she reflected back on these conversations. "I guess I was afraid to confront the surgeon one-on-one," she said. She still wasn't sure exactly why she hadn't told him her foot felt better. "I guess I just didn't want to deal directly with him. He had such a frosty and assertive way about him. And I also really wanted to believe that he knew best."

Lisa underwent the operation. The surgeon removed the bone spur and the ganglion cyst and then fused the arthritic joint, inserting two small titanium screws so that there would be no motion that could cause pain. The day after the procedure, the surgeon called Lisa and said that the postoperative X-ray was "not satisfactory." It looked as if the screws weren't correctly aligned, so Lisa underwent a second operation.

We spoke with Lisa some four months later. "I have pain in my foot all the time," she said. "It has thrown off my gait. So now I also have pain in my hip." It was difficult to stand while teaching; all her household chores had to be delegated to her husband and daughter: shopping, laundry, standing in line in the post office to mail a package. Lisa Norton was frustrated, bitter, and consumed with regret.

Carl Simpson was also a distance runner. As a tall, lanky youth with a fierce, competitive spirit, he grew up scaling the hills of coal country in western Pennsylvania. Then, as a businessman who traveled in the United States and overseas, he never failed to make time for an intense morning run. Simpson, like many athletes, wore down his knees. And like Lisa Norton, he had a bad outcome from surgery. Yet he has no regrets.

Carl was in his early forties when he first developed pain in his left knee. He had been sprinting up steep hills to maintain his conditioning, determined to sustain his times despite the onset of middle age. But after several months, he couldn't ignore the discomfort; the pain worsened, flaring when he ran not only on hills, but also on flat terrain. Carl saw an orthopedic surgeon who told him that the cartilage in the knee was frayed. The surgeon did an arthroscopic procedure in which he threaded a thin fiber-optic device under the kneecap to visualize the joint and remove the torn pieces of cartilage.

"I had an excellent result," Carl told us. "And within a few weeks, I was back running hills."

Eight years and many miles later, Carl again developed pain, this time in his right knee. Every time he straightened his leg, he heard a crunching sound. "I could not even get out of the car without sharp pain," Carl recalled. "And at three in the morning, I had to ask myself, Do I really want to get up to pee?"

He returned to the orthopedic surgeon who had done the previous operation on his other knee and described his intense pain. "I'm ready for surgery again," Carl said.

The doctor studied an X-ray of Carl's knee on his computer screen. "You know, there was much more good cartilage in the other knee when I operated," the doctor explained. "This knee is very degenerated. There are places where it's bone on bone. So arthroscopic surgery may not help." The doctor turned the screen toward Carl and showed him the X-ray images. He could see the stark scalloped edges of the bones nearly touching. The findings in Simpson's knee are typical of aging, where the wear and tear on the joints erode the cartilage until the surfaces of the bones are exposed.

"First, we should try a conservative approach," the orthopedist advised Carl. "It doesn't work for everyone, but it may work for you. I'll write you a prescription for physical therapy, and you may get some relief by taking an anti-inflammatory medication." The surgeon continued, "If it doesn't work, we'll talk again about surgery."

The orthopedist wanted to assess Carl's level of pain and limitation, what some doctors would call Carl's "misery index." The term originated in economics, where it refers to the sum of the unemployment rate and inflation rate, a measure of a nation's financial ill health. In medicine it is used to mean how much pain and limitation a person is experiencing from a condition. Different people have different thresholds of pain; some can tolerate discomfort without it significantly altering the quality of their lives, while others are made miserable by it. Carl Simpson was suffering considerably, and his misery index would be scored as high.

George Loewenstein of Carnegie Mellon University, who has done extensive studies in decision making, distinguishes between "hot" and "cold" emotional states. For example, if we go grocery shopping when we're very hungry, a "hot" emotional state, we tend to buy much more than we need. Similarly, when we're in pain, anxious, angry, or frustrated, we are "hot" and prone to make choices that we imagine will quickly improve our condition. In such a hot state, studies show, patients tend to choose poorly. They discount too deeply the risks a treatment entails, and they overestimate its chances for success. In essence, by recommending conservative measures and a longer period of observation, the surgeon helped to lower Carl's emotional temperature. Not surprisingly, decision making is more deliberate and deep when we have "cooled down," meaning we're more physically comfortable. We're better able to see the downsides as well as the positives and to appreciate the likely impact of a particular choice more accurately.

But after two months of conservative measures, Carl's misery index had hardly budged. He returned to the surgeon, who ordered an MRI of the knee, and then they met again to discuss options.

"I can't even climb the steps in my house without severe pain," Carl said. "I want it fixed, as best as you can."

But Carl told us that before he makes any final decision, he wants to see the numbers. He asked the surgeon for statistics about the risks and benefits of different treatments. And he said that one of the reasons he trusted this surgeon was that the doctor gave him those numbers, providing printouts of clinical studies that compared conservative measures with invasive procedures.

"I just couldn't see how more physical therapy was going to help," he said. "The cartilage was pretty badly frayed. I heard that crunching sound every time I extended my leg. All the physical therapy in the world wasn't going to do anything for that as far as I was concerned. I had tried it for two months and it didn't work."

"There is just so much I can do here," the surgeon told Carl. "At the point when there is bone on bone, we are limited in what we can offer." Carl appreciated his surgeon's honesty but felt that he had arrived at his only option. He didn't hesitate or seek "natural remedies"; he went ahead with the surgery.

"My days as a runner are finished," he told us some months after the operation. "My surgery was not successful. I'm still having significant pain in my knee." The surgeon suggested injections with a new treatment, a resurfacing material that was being tried in cases like Carl's but was still unproven. To date, two such injections had failed to improve Carl's condition. But despite the poor outcome, Carl told us that he had nothing to regret.

In surgery, less than perfect results are hardly rare. Sometimes, falling short of perfection has only a minor impact on a person's life: mild residual discomfort or a keloid scar that detracts from an otherwise successful procedure. At other times, the imperfect result is more problematic. Even with a highly skilled surgeon and outstanding nursing in an excellent hospital, a patient is not guaranteed a good outcome. "I can do everything right," one orthopedist told us, "and the patient can be left with pain and limited use of the joint." You explicitly acknowledge this when you sign a consent form before an operation, verifying that you have read, understood, and asked about the many possible negative outcomes, both minor and major, that fill the document. In effect, you are signing on to uncertainty.

Both Lisa and Carl signed such documents, and both were left in pain after their operations. What, then, might account for deep regret in one case and not the other?

Regret is painful and can be long-lasting, draining a sense of happiness from life. Early studies in the field of regret were conducted by Amos Tversky and Daniel Kahneman, researchers at the Hebrew University in Jerusalem, whose seminal work has informed much of modern cognitive psychology. They examined this issue with regard to money. In one experiment, they asked their research subjects to imagine the feelings of two different investors. The scenario went as follows: A stock falls in price after an "active" investor had recently purchased shares, while another "passive" investor had simply retained the stock in his portfolio. The vast majority of people, more than 90 percent, judged that the active investor would experience more regret because of his recent purchase. Bad outcomes from a recent intervention, Tversky and Kahneman concluded, are more regretted than similar outcomes from passive waiting.

Although these experiments involved investing, they provide insight into medical decisions. Cognitive psychologists like Terry Connolly of the University of Arizona have confirmed the observation that when a person actively chooses a treatment and the outcome is poor, he or she can feel a deeper sense of self-blame and persistent regret. Both Lisa and Carl chose active intervention.

Later work by Dutch researchers led by Marcel Zeelenberg suggested that regret associated with active intervention could be modified by preceding events. The researchers studied this by looking at sports. They asked people to assess the regret of a coach who decides to change the roster of players on a team just before the team loses a game. The level of regret varied depending on whether the team was winning or losing before he altered the roster. If the team was winning and the coach changed the players, people expected that he would experience profound regret; but if the team was losing before, and he changed the roster and then lost the game, his regret would be minimal.

The Dutch sports studies may be relevant to Lisa and Carl. Lisa's cortisone injections were working well, and she could enjoy walking with little pain for hours in Paris. This is analogous to the sports team winning. So when she "changed roster"—that is, when she shifted to an extensive surgery rather than staying with the winning strategy of the injection—her team "lost" and her sense of regret was profound. Carl, on the other hand, was on the "losing team," his misery index high and prolonged. Physical therapy was not alleviating his pain and immobility, so when his operation did not succeed either, he did not feel much regret. This is one possible contributor to why Lisa but not Carl experienced regret.

Of course, Lisa's winning strategy may or may not have been a good long-term option. A third cortisone shot might not have been effective. Following the sports analogy, the score then changed and the team began to lose. At that point, shifting strategy would be expected to result in less regret, even if at the end of the "game" her team lost, meaning the operation was not a success.

In considering clinical choices, cognitive psychologists have described what is termed "omission bias." Some people prefer not to actively choose a treatment because they fear the greater regret they will experience from committing to a treatment if there is a bad outcome, especially a side effect. This anticipation of regret may lead some patients to avoid ("omit") rather than take ("commit to") a treatment.

This "omission bias" has been invoked to explain the low rate of vaccination for illnesses like influenza, typically 35 to 45 percent of adults. While people are feeling good, they anticipate the regret they would experience if they got sick from the injection. Even though the risks of side effects from the vaccine are low and typically very mild, many people prefer to omit the vaccination and take the risk of later developing influenza, which generally has more severe effects on the body. Not surprisingly, those who later catch a bad flu then regret that they omitted the vaccination and may blame themselves for being shortsighted.

Terry Connolly and his team of researchers at the University of Arizona found that when there is a negative outcome after treatment, the target of regret may be the decision process preceding the choice. This was the case with Lisa after her failed surgery. She repeatedly trawled over the events, the sequence of conversations with doctors and family and friends, as well as the shifts in her own mind-set, looking for what she could have changed.

Connolly distinguishes between "normal" and "nonstandard" decision processes. The latter deviate from an individual's usual logic, behavior, or preferences. Lisa had had the experience of her lupus, where she followed her naturalism orientation, spending months in bed reading books that proposed alternative approaches to autoimmune diseases. Ultimately, when the lupus did not improve, she decided to pursue mainstream remedies, including drugs with significant side effects. She sought second opinions and felt that she had a clear view of her options. Equally important, Lisa felt that her rheumatologist understood her mind-set. "He knew where I was coming from, that I hated those drugs and wanted to come off them as soon as possible," she said. In essence, the doctor molded his approach to fit Lisa's, trying repeatedly to decrease the amount of medication she took, only to find that her lupus flared when she was prescribed the lower doses. It took several years before she went into remission, but despite her frustration with what she termed a "roller-coaster ride" of diminished doses followed by intensive treatment, with all the side effects of insomnia, voracious appetite, and swollen body parts, she never regretted the decisions she'd made along the way. With her lupus, she followed her "normal" process. But with her foot surgery, Lisa realized that she had abandoned it.

Before her trip to Europe, she felt she'd entered into a "negotiation" with the doctor. It was a different type of negotiation from the one Dr. Carter told us he conducts with his patients, where he explores what a person wants or doesn't want and why. "The doctor agreed to give me the cortisone injection so long as I scheduled the surgery for the week I returned," Lisa told us. She felt that if she changed her mind, she would be backing out of a promise she had made. "I really don't know why I let myself be boxed in," she said. "I felt I sort of owed him something in the way we had agreed to go forward."

Many patients have such feelings and don't want to disappoint their doctors. Psychologist Judith Hall at Northeastern University and health researcher Debra Roter at Johns Hopkins have extensively studied physician-patient interactions. They focused on the emotions that patients often feel in what is typically a power imbalance—the doctor is an authority figure with special knowledge and skill, the patient needs expert assistance to remedy a problem. Many patients fear appearing "difficult," worried that they will alienate the doctor by questioning his thinking and challenging his advice. One patient we spoke with who was contemplating hip surgery even worried that his pointed questions could cause his doctor to do a less than excellent job for him, "subconsciously taking his annoyance out on me." This scenario prevented the patient from discussing his concerns candidly with his doctor, even though there was no indication the physician was anything less than professional. Moreover, when a physician expresses disapproval or dislike of a patient's thinking or feelings, Hall and Roter found, the patient often blames herself, imagining the doctor's judgment pinpoints a flaw in the patient's character. "I didn't want to be a curmudgeon type of patient," Lisa told us. "And I can be that way, resisting what the doctor recommends."

So, she explained, "I was afraid to confront the doctor one-on-one. I think I wanted someone else to tell him about my concerns." The nurse and her school principal had rightly advised Lisa to tell the doctor herself. "I was being a total chicken about it. I just didn't want to deal directly with him."

Even a strong-minded and well-informed person like Lisa may find it difficult to exercise her usual degree of autonomy when she's ill. We spoke with a renowned professor of English at a prestigious university who is used to prevailing in faculty debates and in negotiations with the college president. He fractured his leg and underwent a series of risky operations. "Each time I sat with the surgeon, it was as if my mind went out the window," the professor told us. "I was like a frightened child in front of him and couldn't think at all."

When considering an important medical decision, patients are often advised to obtain a second opinion. Lisa sought a second opinion from another prominent orthopedic surgeon. "When I asked him what was best," Lisa told us, "he turned the question back on me, asking, 'What do you want?' So I asked my second-opinion surgeon what he would recommend if I were his mother."

Patients have often asked us the same question that Lisa posed to the orthopedic surgeon: "What would you do for your mother, your sister, or even for yourself?" This query is essentially asking, "Tell me what you really think is 'best.'" The patient wants the physician to forget malpractice, cost, professional relationships, hospital affiliations, and anything else that might limit or influence his or her advice about treatment. But even with the same clinical problem, what is best for the surgeon's mother might not be best for Lisa.

Our two mothers, in fact, had taken very different approaches to medical problems. One mother was a deep doubter and a minimalist; she had no place for authoritarian injunctions and recoiled when a doctor, with the best intentions, stated plainly what he thought she should do. The other, a maximalist and a believer in science and technology, profoundly respectful of the medical profession, would tell us, "The doctor said to do this, so I do it." She never missed a pill, never resisted a procedure, certain that each recommendation was one step closer to regaining health. So the answer to Lisa's question depends on several assumptions.

The first is that the mind-set and preferences of the doctor's mother are the same as those of the patient who is asking the question. The second assumption is that there is a clear best option that every expert would agree upon.

Very often in medicine there is more than one way to address a problem. As we noted previously, much of medicine is still an uncertain science, existing in a gray zone—not clearly black or white. In Lisa's case, some physicians might have advised her not to fuse the joint, leaving that as a later option should it be needed. Others would assert, as Lisa's doctor did, that fusion clearly was required. Medical journals regularly feature articles that explore the differences in experts' judgments about cases where there is no clear "best" approach. These kinds of complex and controversial cases are the regular focus of clinical conferences, where specialists discuss and debate the merits of different approaches.

We have no way to know what treatment was best for Lisa. In fact, from the outset there was uncertainty about the nature of her problem. "The surgeon gave me these vague responses when what I wanted was a clear weighing of how each of the problems in my foot, the bone spur, the ganglion cyst, the arthritis in the joint, contributed to my pain," Lisa said. Of course, this kind of clarity is often impossible to achieve. Only after removing one or two or all three of these abnormalities could a more exact answer be given. That kind of uncertainty pervades much of medical decision making. And in situations where one can't predict the outcome accurately, how the decision is made can be as important as what decision is made.

Lisa told us, "In this case, I wanted the ganglion cyst removed. And I wanted the bone spur removed. But I started getting really nervous about the fusion. If the foot doesn't have a spur sticking into the joint anymore, if the ganglion cyst is removed, maybe the arthritis wouldn't be that bad, maybe the joint would calm down." This was her logic. "But I also wanted to believe that he was really on the right track and that he was going to fix my problem. I said to myself, Okay, you are going into surgery anyway, and I guess he knows best. So I listened to what he said. I usually advocate well for myself, but in this case, I did not.

"I should have erred on the conservative side," she continued, "because the body has a powerful mechanism for healing itself." Here, she was expressing her underlying naturalism orientation. Then she revealed a "minimalism" orientation as well. "My general philosophy about medicine is to do the least possible," she told us.

It is often suggested to bring a friend or family member or patient advocate to the appointment to serve as another set of "eyes and ears," better able to capture what the physician is saying. In Lisa's case, such a companion could also have been the "mouth," to articulate what Lisa had difficulty expressing. She knew what she wanted to say but couldn't bring herself to say it. Of course, the companion needs to both understand and represent your mind-set.

Similarly, second opinions can be very helpful when patients face uncertain or serious medical diagnoses. But in Lisa's case, the second surgeon seemed to be overly influenced by another prominent imperative in modern medical culture: patient autonomy. Lisa told us that the doctor said, "'You can do it, or you can wait.' He just wasn't being helpful. He kept saying, 'It's all up to you.'" As the University of

Michigan's Carl Schneider has shown, the principle of autonomy may be taken too far in some instances and for certain patients, where the doctor exempts himself from his role as guide and puts the burden of choice entirely on the patient's shoulders. This may have been the case with Lisa's second opinion: Do whatever you want. Arizona's Connolly notes that as patients achieve greater autonomy in decision making, they run a greater risk of regret; if the outcome is poor, the patient can end up blaming herself. Of course, this is a delicate balance, because in the face of a bad outcome, a person may also regret not exercising enough autonomy. And this, it appeared, was the case with Lisa.

Lisa Norton told us she hoped her story would help others making difficult decisions. She felt she had betrayed her own instincts and, in effect, failed to follow her normal process.

What about Carl Simpson? He was also deeply disappointed with the outcome of his operation. Marcel Zeelenberg distinguishes between regret and disappointment. Disappointment is an unavoidable aspect of making difficult choices: Sometimes the results fall short of what we had hoped for. But disappointment carries none of the self-blame that typically marks regret. Carl felt fully satisfied with how he had made his decision. "I'm a little bit of a pain in the rear end," he said with a laugh. "I ask a lot of questions. My surgeon knows how my mind works, and he gave me answers."

As Northeastern's Judith Hall has observed, a doctor who successfully advises a patient facing uncertain choices must enter into the patient's mind. "A doctor should encourage the patient, prompt him to explore his feelings and preferences," Hall said. However, as we noted earlier, doctors usually aren't formally trained in how to elicit a person's preferences, either in medical school or during their residency. And as we have seen, doctors sometimes unwittingly project their own biases and preferences onto their patients.

"Do I regret what I did?" Carl asked rhetorically. "No."

Carl had followed his way of approaching problems. And although he has persistent and limiting pain in his left knee, "I knew I did everything that could be done, and I did it right." Researchers on regret would say Carl's process was "normal."

The optimal process has been termed "shared medical decision making" between doctor and patient. After together reviewing information about risks and benefits of treatment options, doctor and patient then customize the care according to the mind-set and orientation of the patient. Sharing the decision with a doctor who understands your preferences means sharing the burden of choice, so you lessen your risk for regret.

Five

Neighborly Advice

Prostate cancer is among the most commonly diagnosed malignancies. In 2010, more than two hundred thousand American men learned that they have the tumor. Making the diagnosis by a biopsy is relatively easy. But once the diagnosis is made, choosing treatment, if any, is hardly straightforward.

Matt Conlin, a venture capitalist in Chicago, glanced down and checked his BlackBerry. He had four new messages. Three were birthday greetings from friends—he had turned sixty-six that week. The fourth was a message from his secretary to call his doctor back.

Two weeks before, Matt had seen a urologist because he'd started to feel the need to urinate so urgently that he sometimes had to break away from business meetings to get to the men's room. But by the time he arrived for his appointment, the symptom had subsided. After examining Matt, the urologist said, "I'm not sure why you had such frequent urination. You have the prostate of a young man." The urologist looked over the blood tests that had been done by his internist. He noted that Matt's prostate-specific antigen, or PSA, had risen slightly, from 2.8 to 3.0. "I really think that small bump in the PSA is nothing," the urologist had said, "but the only way to be absolutely sure is to do an ultrasound with a biopsy." He went on to say, "We don't have to do this now. We could wait another few months, repeat the PSA, and then decide."

"In my world, information is power," replied Matt. "Let's do it now." The biopsy took less than fifteen minutes and was not particularly painful. The urologist told Matt that on the ultrasound study his prostate gland looked entirely normal. "I really don't think you have anything to worry about."

Matt put away his BlackBerry. He had another meeting in ten minutes. A computer software company in India was seeking more capital to expand its operations. Ten minutes should be long enough to return the urologist's call.

"I'm really surprised," the doctor said, "but it turns out that there is some cancer in the gland. I didn't expect this." The doctor tried to reassure him, saying that only three of the twelve biopsies contained small amounts of tumor, all on the left side of his prostate gland. He gave Matt a number—6—a Gleason score, a measure of the tumor's aggressiveness. "It's in the midrange, not the worst at all."

"I was unnerved by that call from the urologist," Matt told us. "It was bad enough to hear that I had cancer, but the shock was much greater after being reassured by the doctor that my prostate felt normal, that the ultrasound study was normal, too, and that the rise in

PSA was nothing. This was not supposed to happen. My trust and confidence in this physician were completely shaken."

As physicians, we recognize that we often walk a fine line with our patients, trying to allay their anxiety and concern by giving reassurances that are based largely on probabilities. We spoke with other patients whose doctors had initially assured them that their symptoms or physical examination didn't suggest a serious underlying disease, only to have those assurances proven wrong. A forty-five-year-old teacher had been told by two specialists based on physical examination and an ultrasound study that a small nodule in her neck was "almost certainly" benign; however, a biopsy showed thyroid cancer. A sixty-two-year-old physician and marathon runner developed indigestion. His internist performed a complete physical examination, told him everything was fine, and prescribed an acid blocker. A month later, he was rushed to the hospital and underwent open heart surgery to bypass four blocked coronary arteries; the "indigestion" was really a symptom of heart disease. A twenty-six-year-old writer was found to have a minimal elevation in one of her liver function tests at her yearly checkup. Her doctor told her, "Don't worry about it. One glass of wine can do that." Although there is a long list of trivial causes of slightly elevated liver tests, in her case, follow-up and an eventual liver biopsy showed extensive inflammation from hepatitis C infection.

No physician is right all the time. Every physician is wrong sometime. Perfection is impossible. How does the patient react to that reality? When we as physicians were wrong in the past, some of our patients left us. They could no longer trust our judgment. Doubt clouded every conversation. Uncertainty shadowed every subsequent recommendation. Confidence in the physician helps a patient cope with the vicissitudes of his illness; trust in the doctor reduces fear and allays the sense of vulnerability. These patients, looking to restore this sense of confidence, decided to seek a new doctor. On the other hand, we've been surprised by patients who didn't leave after an error but used the mistake as a paradoxical strategy for more attentive care. One man we both cared for said after we acknowledged our mistake and apologized to him, "Now I believe you'll pay extra-special attention to my case, because you're so worried that you might be wrong again in the future."

It's easy to acknowledge the truth of physician fallibility in the abstract; it's much more difficult to accept it when you actually experience it, when your own doctor's soothing words turn out to be wrong. It can shake the foundations of your confidence like an earthquake; the ground you stand on can no longer support you. The experience of how a diagnosis is made, what doctors thought and said, can have a profound impact on how you apply their advice about treatment. Indeed, both of us as patients had this experience where our physicians proved fallible. Someone who is already a doubter is reinforced in that mind-set. A believer struggles to maintain his or her sense of belief as the seeds of doubt are planted.

Matt Conlin never had any reason to doubt a physician's advice before. He had never been seriously ill and prided himself on his youthful physique and energy. Medically, everything had always gone according to plan for him. He had had an EKG and colonoscopy, both normal. His blood pressure and cholesterol were checked regularly, and when his doctor noted a slightly elevated cholesterol, he prescribed a statin. The physician assured him he would tolerate it well, and he did; soon his cholesterol had dropped as predicted. But now the world of medicine looked very different. The stark reality of uncertainty was in the foreground of his vision.

M att Conlin designated one of his senior analysts to sit in for
him on the meeting about the investment in India. Then he
told his secretary to hold all calls and closed his office door. When an
investment turned sour, Matt went back and looked at the numbers
himself, to understand the problem and try to solve it. Now he told
himself that he needed to find the numbers, to rely on his own information. He began a Google search on prostate cancer.

"If you Google 'prostate cancer,'" he told us, "you get millions of
hits." Using the same methodical strategy that he applied to investments, he started with general background information before delving
into the specifics. He went to the Web sites of mainstream organizations like the National Cancer Institute and the American Cancer
Society. All presented three options: surgery, radiation, or no immediate treatment but close monitoring, so-called watchful waiting. Each
approach was outlined in broad language without indicating which
was superior. He wanted more details on treatment, so he began to
read medical articles. "I was looking for differences that might be important for me," Matt told us. After a few hours in front of the screen,
he was overwhelmed. "The technical terms were confusing and there
was too much information. I didn't know how to interpret what I was
reading. Where did my case fit? I was looking for more guidance. So
I went to Barnes and Noble and bought an armful of books on prostate cancer."

One of the books was written by a prominent urologist in another city who stated that he had one of the highest rates of cure and
lowest incidence of complications in the United States.

Matt called this urologist's office. The receptionist began to take
down his information, but after getting his name and date of birth, she

abruptly halted the conversation. "I'm sorry, but we have a cutoff of sixty-five years old," she said. "You're sixty-six."

Matt was taken aback. How could there be such a rigid age cutoff? "Last week, I was sixty-five," he replied. "So if I had called last week before my sixty-sixth birthday, then I could have gotten an appointment?"

"Yes, that's our rule."

Matt had accumulated not only considerable wealth over the course of decades, but also considerable contacts among powerful figures in business and politics. He returned to his computer and searched the list of trustees of the hospital where the urologist practiced. He quickly found the name of a man he invested with. A phone call later, Matt heard back from the doctor's office. "They said I could come in whenever it was convenient. Apparently, I was now an excellent candidate for surgery," he told us.

Matt flew out to see this surgeon, who explained that he performed a traditional operation, a so-called open procedure, rather than using a laparoscope with robotic assistance. "In my hands, it's the best way to a cure, and I can see the nerves clearly and preserve them so you won't become impotent." In the past, Matt would have been impressed by the surgeon's confidence. But he thought back to the urologist who had assured him that everything would be fine, that he didn't have cancer. So now he had doubts. He wasn't ready to commit to this surgery yet. He would explore other options, like robotic surgery or radiation.

It wasn't difficult for him to secure an appointment with a well-known radiation specialist. After sitting for nearly two hours in a waiting room decorated with several photos of local celebrities, each inscribed with thanks to the doctor, he was evaluated by a medical student who took his history and performed a rectal examination. Next, a resident came and did the same. "So after these young doctors examine me, the boss comes into the examination room and says he wants to do yet another digital rectal exam. I had now had four normal prostate examinations in the last month, two of them in the last twenty minutes. And I have the images from the normal ultrasound study in my hand." It had been nearly three hours since Matt had arrived at the office. "I told him I really preferred not to have yet another rectal exam. I came here to discuss treatment options. But he said that if I didn't want a digital exam, I might as well leave. I considered going, but since I had invested this much time already, I let him do the examination. Again, normal.

"The specialist then casually flipped through my pile of records and said, 'You know, for anyone of your age who wants to keep his sexual function intact, radiation is really the way to go. Surgeons will tell you they can spare the nerves, but even with robotic surgery it often doesn't work.'

"I was really annoyed by this visit, and I was totally uninterested in spending any more time in that office," Matt said. "But that didn't mean that radiation was necessarily out." He had learned as an investor not to make decisions in the heat of the moment. "I looked at the photos on the way out—clearly he was the top guy. I needed to give it more thought.

"Proton beam popped up in my research," Matt continued.

Proton beam therapy uses a special kind of high-energy particle. Doctors who offered the treatment contended that you could focus the high-energy beam more accurately than with classical forms of radiation. The focused radiation theoretically was better able to spare the healthy surrounding tissues and eradicate the cancer in the gland with less toxicity. Only a few hospitals around the country had the technology to deliver this kind of radiation.

"It seemed elegant, just the kind of nuanced difference I was looking for," Matt said. "I called a friend, and he put me in touch with one of his business partners who was treated with proton beam. When I called the man, it turned out that not only was he treated there, but he had been involved in the start-up financing. He just raved about it."

Matt Conlin was trained as an engineer before entering finance, and this background began to guide much of his thinking. Here, he told us, was a precise, controlled beam that would reduce as much as possible the risks of the radiation. "It made sense to me." So he prepared himself to relocate to a medical center with a proton beam unit in Southern California. "It seems like I have contacts everywhere, and I wasn't shy about using them. An associate there had a guesthouse and a car. I would take the treatment when it was bitter cold in Chicago, and it would be perfect weather in California. The more I imagined it, the more pleasant it seemed." But then Matt checked himself in order to avoid the kind of error that people often make in investments—consider the long-term downsides, not just the immediate returns.

"I read more and learned that even with proton beam, problems can creep up over time, like bowel incontinence and impotence, just like with standard radiation treatment," he said. "I didn't want to take the chance of later damage, although I did like the idea of a nonsurgical procedure."

Matt said that, without exaggeration, he spoke with more than twenty different physicians expert in the field of prostate cancer. He was determined to find that subtle difference, to identify the advantage for him that must exist in one of the treatments at a certain medical center or with a specific doctor or technology.

But he was beginning to tire in his search. "I figured by then if I went to a surgeon, he was going to cut. If I went to a radiation specialist, he was going to radiate. And each specialist recommended their own way of doing it and gave me these statistics. But the numbers were not helping me."

Would Bernoulli's formula, multiplying the probability of an outcome by its utility, give Matt the numbers he sought to make a rational decision? Let's assume that surgery and radiation give a roughly equal chance of cure. Given that assumption, we need consider only the side effects. We need to know the probability of each side effect for each treatment and the impact (in numerical form) it would have on Matt's life. First, we would do the calculation for surgery, and then we would repeat the calculation for radiation treatment. The most rational choice for Matt would be the treatment that provides the highest expected utility. This would be the treatment that avoids the worst side effects and has the least negative impact on his life.

Alan Schwartz and George Bergus, professors at the University of Illinois and University of Iowa, respectively, vividly illustrate the daunting challenge of doing this calculation in their primer *Medical Decision Making*. They use as an example an informed consent document given to men considering prostate surgery. The document lists eleven different potential adverse outcomes, including common ones like erectile dysfunction and incontinence with leakage of urine, as well as less common ones like clots in the legs after surgery, infections, the need for repeat operations, and so on. The list of eleven outcomes doesn't even include the potential risks of anesthesia. Schwartz and Bergus calculated that for these eleven potential side effects, there are over two thousand combinations. The next step is to imagine the quality of your life with each of these two thousand combinations of side effects and assign a number for each.

Recognizing how overwhelming this prospect is, some experts suggest that patients should focus only on the most frequent adverse outcomes. But even by winnowing the list of major side effects of prostate surgery to urinary incontinence and sexual impotence, the patient is still at a loss to assess the impact, since there is a great deal of variability in terms of the severity and duration of each negative outcome. Do you dribble urine only occasionally or do you consistently wet your underwear? Do you have a partial erection or no erection? Is your erection improved with Viagra? And if improved, is it enough for gratifying sexual relations? Or is lovemaking marred by anxious disappointment? Do these side effects last for months, or years, or are they permanent?

For a moment, let's put aside these complexities and see how researchers have devised ways to come up with a number for the "utility" or impact of living with a side effect. One method is a rating scale. Matt would be given a straight line where 0 represents death and 100 represents perfect health. Then he would be asked to designate where being impotent would fall on that line, and a number would be assigned. Similarly, Matt would try to designate where on the line he would fall if he had urinary incontinence, and again a utility number would be assigned.

A second method is termed the "time trade-off." In this approach, you imagine how much you'd be willing to shorten your life in return for perfect health. In this case, Matt would be asked how many years of life he would give up to avoid impotence or incontinence. Using the years of life traded, a utility number is calculated.

A third approach is called the "standard gamble." This method gauges how much risk you're willing to take to avoid a side effect. For example, the doctor would ask Matt to imagine that a "magic pill" is newly arrived from a drug company. The magic medication will prevent a side effect (in this case impotence or incontinence) but is immediately fatal in some people. In Matt's case, what odds would he need to take the gamble? If the pill prevents impotence in 99 percent of patients and is fatal in 1 percent, will he take it? What about 90/10 or 80/20? Once the last acceptable gamble is determined, the odds are used to calculate the utility number in Bernoulli's formula.* However, a wealth of recent research shows that putting a number on the utility or impact of living with a side effect is unreliable. First, current methods for assessing utility are not interchangeable. Numerous studies show that a single patient using the three different methods—the 0 to 100 scale, the time trade-off, the standard gamble—will often come up with different numbers for the same side effect. If all the methods accurately determined the impact of the side effect for that patient, each method should give the same number. Moreover, even the simple scale from 0 to 100 can vary—what is "perfect health"? For whom? For a sixty-year-old or a twenty-year-old? Does it mean you never have a headache or indigestion?

Second, the patient is asked to assess his or her life in the future under unfamiliar conditions. Imagining different scenarios based on written descriptions or listening to a doctor describe a condition cannot be grasped in the same way as actually living it. Dr. Peter Ubel, a professor at Duke University, who has extensively studied patients' utility assessments, notes the "central problem with these methods . . . is that they require respondents [patients] to think about a health state they are not actually experiencing." Even we, as physicians, who have cared for many people who developed side effects from treatments, can't imagine what our lives would be like with those side effects.

For that reason, researchers have tried to get a more accurate assessment of utility by surveying patients who are currently living with a given side effect. In theory, the utility number provided by these patients could be used to guide decision making for those considering treatment options. But the experience of living with that side effect is not static or fixed. It can depend on the person's emotions at the time

---

* For more detail regarding calculating the time trade-off and standard gamble, see the notes.

he is asked. If you ask a patient when he is anxious or in pain to assign a utility number, and later ask him again when he is calm or comfortable, you can get very different answers. People also adapt to their changed life after treatment for a disorder. That adaptation can be highly individual and further fluctuate over time so that a person might score his or her life better, then worse, then better again. Over a period of weeks to months, studies show that patients with conditions as varied as coronary disease and breast cancer assigned values that fluctuated by as much as 50 percent.

We believe these findings argue that the effort to reduce medical decision making to numbers is misconceived and reductionist, overly simplifying a complex and vexing process that is fraught with conflict and emotion.

We live in a culture that looks increasingly to numbers for answers. Numbers communicate a sense of precision in the face of uncertainty. Matt Conlin relied on them in his decisions at work. He was determined to find the numbers that were relevant to his particular case. But despite hours of research and numerous consultations with specialists, he could not. The numbers on quality of life after treatment for prostate cancer reflected averages of thousands of men with all the limitations noted above. He still could not answer the question Where do I, as an individual, fit in?

Matt began to think about his family. His mother died at ninety-three in her sleep. His father died at ninety-seven in an accident, slipping off the roof of his house while repairing shingles. His paternal grandfather, he was told, lived to one hundred five. "I thought that if I am destined to live to ninety-plus, like others in my family—then I need to treat this cancer. Watchful waiting is not for me. I am not likely to die of something else, like a heart attack or stroke, before the cancer could grow and spread." Matt's effort to place his life into the time frame of his parents and grandparents was, in a sense, an availability bias. Their dramatic longevity had been a touchstone all his life. "Furthermore, I have to think long and hard about side effects, because I will have a long time to develop them and live with them." For Matt, that was the problem with radiation, even proton beam. No one could give him the kinds of assurances that he wanted, that he would not develop late side effects. "So," Matt told us, "it should be surgery, because with an operation you could take out all the cancer, and complications occur pretty much immediately. And robotics seemed to make to most sense to me, with my engineering background." Matt was aware that studies did not show a significant difference between robotic surgery and open surgery by an experienced surgeon. "But," he said, "it seemed to me that this robotic technology could eliminate a lot of potential human error. I thought about how any surgeon can have a bad day, and make a mistake on me. A robot would make a mistake less likely." Matt showed what we call a "technology orientation," the view that new science and technology are automatically superior to older approaches, a view that reflected his training as an engineer and his temperament as a venture capitalist investing in new developments. In contrast, those with a naturalism orientation would view the latest technology with suspicion, as being overhyped and not able to deliver on its promise.

With a technology orientation in mind, Matt did "due diligence" on urological surgeons who used robotic methods to remove the prostate gland. He studied the backgrounds of each surgeon the way an investor looks at the pedigree of the CEO before investing in a company. Matt called the surgeon who seemed to have the most experience and best reputation in Chicago and set up an appointment. "When I entered the waiting room, a patient was cheerfully chatting with the nurses. He told me he was back to thank the doctor after the operation." This made a deep impression on Matt. He fantasized that one day he would be the one coming in to thank the surgeon. At the end of his appointment, the doctor suggested that he speak with some of his patients, other men who'd had the surgery. Matt contacted two of them. They seemed satisfied with the results and said they were "fine" within a year. But Matt confessed to us that he didn't push as far as he might in a business investment. He was reluctant to invade their privacy to ask hard questions about their sex lives or whether they leaked urine.

It was some six months after the operation when we spoke again with Matt. "I still drip urine," he said, "particularly when I exercise. Sometimes when I cough or sneeze or twist around quickly to reach something behind me, I go, Oops, there are a few drops. It's really aggravating. And I can't wear khaki trousers. I have a business trip to Switzerland next week, and I like to wear khakis on the flight. But dark stains show up from the urine. So the khakis are retired for the time being."

Matt Conlin was very open with us. "And on the sexual function side, the erections are not strong enough." He tried Viagra, but it didn't consistently help. "Although things seemed to get a bit better as time went on, my erections are still not adequate, not at all what they were before. But you know," Matt reflected, "I'm serious. If the doctor or one of his patients asked me how I was now, I would say I was 110 percent. So I wonder if those two men I spoke to before the surgery and even the guy in the waiting room really were 'fine.'"

This disconnect between the truth and what Matt would say coincides with the results from studies that compared how men reported side effects after prostate surgery to their surgeons with their statements to a neutral interviewer obtaining answers in the privacy of their home. What accounts for this discrepancy? Reports of side effects are often colored by the desire to please the physician and express thanks for removing the cancer. Other times, men may want to minimize their distress by compartmentalizing it, a common coping mechanism. One patient said to us, "I tell everyone I feel better than I do, and that makes me feel better."

Even when physicians receive accurate reports of side effects, research has shown that doctors assess the impact of side effects after prostate surgery very differently from the men who have had the operation. The same disconnect between physician and patient is true for radiation treatments as well. What seems minor to many doctors is often a major source of frustration and unhappiness for the patient. Studies also show that when doctors advise patients about which treatment to choose, they project their own biases with regard to the impact of side effects on quality of life. Surgeons focus on unacceptable side effects of radiation, while radiation therapists emphasize the unacceptable side effects of surgery. We saw this phenomenon of "projection bias" with the doctor who advised Patrick Baptiste to have radioactive iodine rather than surgery. The physician's advice was framed to minimize the side effects of the treatment he'd recommended and accentuate the side effects of the other possible treatments.

We wondered, after all his research and deliberation, if Matt Conlin regretted his decision to have robotic surgery.

"Well, I'm thrilled that my PSA is zero," he said. "There is no better number as far as I am concerned." Indeed, studies show that if Matt stays at zero, his cancer won't recur. "There is nothing more that I could have done—no point in looking back. In fact, a few weeks after the surgery, I threw out my files on prostate cancer. It's time to move forward."

While Matt Conlin was recovering from his operation in Chicago, some two thousand miles away in West Los Angeles, Steven Baum, a sixty-two-year-old clinical psychologist, received a message to call his urologist. Steven had known for several years that he had a large prostate gland, and the urologist who cared for him had reassured him that his apparently high PSA level, when corrected for the size of the prostate, was not actually high at all. He had seen the urologist two weeks earlier because routine blood work showed the PSA had risen by a full point. "He examined me and said everything was fine." As before, the doctor felt that the large prostate explained the increase in the PSA level. Although he said there was no cause for concern, the urologist recommended a biopsy "to be sure." "I don't think you're going to have any problem. Don't worry about it."

Steven Baum returned the call. "Well, we found some growths—the pathologist classified most of this as a 6, but there was a very small amount of 7," the urologist said, "and I'm concerned about the 7."

Steven had no idea what the numbers meant. The urologist elaborated: "Most of this is run-of-the-mill stuff, we don't worry too much about it. But come in and we'll talk." Later, Steven told us, "I'm listening to him, trying to figure out what he is really saying. Do I have cancer? And what is 6 and 7?"

He said that he was able to block out the conversation with the doctor from his mind until he finished seeing his last patient, shortly before seven p.m. And then it all came back full force. He tried to maintain a sense of calm. "But then I looked on the Internet and started getting very anxious. It sounded to me like this was cancer. This was serious."

Steven met with the urologist the next day. He brought his wife to the appointment. The doctor spoke with confidence: "You have a very little bit of aggressive tumor, but we will get it all out with surgery. I wouldn't recommend radiation for you because your gland is too big."

"Before he brought it up, I was already worried about side effects," Steven told us, "but the urologist told me, 'You are not going to have any side effects. It's all going to be fine.' The urologist went on to say that 'after thirty years of doing this operation, I have perfected my technique. I have the best results in Los Angeles. My assistant will contact you to set a date for your surgery.'"

The urologist stood up to escort Steven and his wife to the door. But after a few steps, Steven stopped abruptly and asked, "What do I do about my anxiety?"

The doctor nodded sympathetically. "I can schedule you in two weeks. We'll be finished with it."

Baum told us how he left the appointment feeling strangely elated. "I said to myself, Oh, my God, this is going to be fine. It's a great relief to go from thinking I'm dying tomorrow to hearing that the operation has no serious side effects because the doctor has done it so well so many times, and that I'll come out as good as new." Steven's wife, also a psychologist, was similarly swept away. "She said, 'Well, if I had a prostate, I would want this operation, too.'"

Steven, an energetic man with a full head of curly hair, a ruddy complexion, and a ready laugh, was keen to talk about his interactions with doctors and the insights he had gleaned from trying to choose a treatment. "As a psychologist, I'm trained to have experiences and then to look at my experiences and be able to see clearly what's happening to me. Certainly if I'm so confused, so overwhelmed, doing and thinking things that I never expected, it might be useful to others to hear my story."

After his diagnosis, Steven told us that he initially had "bizarre" and unrealistic thoughts. "I thought, Maybe I don't really have cancer. Maybe the laboratory mixed up my biopsy with someone else's. I just couldn't believe I was going through this." Steven's "bizarre thoughts" are not uncommon. People often feel a sense of unreality and denial when receiving an unexpected and serious diagnosis. Steven Baum's "bizarre" thinking also has some connection with fact. When he had searched the Internet, he found a recommendation that patients should always get a second opinion from a certified pathologist on the biopsy. Indeed, pathologists can differ on the Gleason score, some interpreting the findings differently despite the same uniform criteria.

Steven explained: "When you feel so insecure, you want someone who is stronger than you are—a powerful person who is going to make it all go away. As psychologists, we look at the doctor as a parent figure. What he is essentially saying is, 'I'm going to take care of you.'"

Steven understood from his training the tension between the desire to believe and the need to doubt. "More than anything else, you want a savior, someone to hold you. It goes way back to when you were a child, wanting a parent to say it's all going to be okay. And my urologist was saying that. So a part of me was saying, 'I want him to take care of me. Everything will be fine.'" Then he checked himself. "But the other part of me was saying, 'Are you a fool?' I've had three strikes with him. He told me three times that everything was okay, that the prostate gland was big but had no growth, that the high PSA level was not meaningful given the size of the gland, and the biopsy was not really necessary and would be negative." Steven Baum, like Matt Conlin, was unnerved by having received repeated reassurances that turned out to be wrong.

But unlike Matt Conlin, who considers himself "a numbers person," Steven Baum, by his own account, is not. He did not immerse himself in data. Rather, as an outgoing and social man, with what he called "an amazing network of people" in Los Angeles, "I decided to delay the surgery and started talking to everyone I knew about prostate cancer." He felt no hesitation in telling friends and colleagues that he had been diagnosed with prostate cancer, to connect with other men who had the same condition, and to draw from their personal experiences. Steven found that an older psychiatrist with whom he'd trained had been diagnosed with prostate cancer and had begun a blog to detail his experiences. This older man had had radiation therapy, and then several years later the cancer recurred. Now he was receiving hormonal therapy to treat the metastases. "You can live with it, Steve. It's not a death warrant," his former mentor told him. Another of his mentors, also diagnosed with prostate cancer, chose watchful waiting and was doing well. He recommended that Steven seek a second opinion with his doctor at a different hospital nearby.

"My father died at that hospital," Steven told us. "So my unconscious voice was telling me, 'You go there to die.' I realized that kind of stuff is not really pertinent, that just because my father died there doesn't mean that the doctor and the care at that hospital would not be excellent."

Using his "network," Steven found a urologist who was expert at laparoscopic robotic surgery, the procedure that Matt Conlin ultimately chose. This doctor laid out in stark terms the pros and cons of the different surgeries. He pointed out that a recent analysis comparing traditional open surgery with laparoscopic prostatectomy concluded that the side effects of impotence and incontinence were essentially the same with both. The main advantage, he contended, was that the recovery time was faster with a robotic procedure. "He just gave me the facts, no reassurances," said Steven. "He was very much the opposite of the first urologist.

"In fact, he was brutally honest—he said there is about a 50 percent chance of getting erectile dysfunction. And at that point I thought, What the hell is erectile dysfunction? Does that mean you will never have an erection again? Does that mean that you are only a little soft but still can make love?"

Steven Baum said that in psychology, you learn never to assume that you heard the "message" correctly. "It's the notion that someone is telling you one thing, but you are hearing another. When he said 50 percent of men get erectile dysfunction, my assumption was that 50 percent will never have sex again in their lives. I really like sex, and my wife also really likes sex. It's a big part of our life."

Steven had identified an important gap in communication between doctor and patient. The language and terms used by physicians can mean something quite different to a patient or have no clear meaning at all. This has been highlighted in studies of many disorders. With regard to prostate cancer, a team of experts led by Dr. Timothy Wilt at the University of Minnesota reviewed more than seven hundred papers in an effort to determine which therapy was superior and caused the fewest side effects. They could not conclude that surgery, radiation, or watchful waiting was clearly best for men with prostate cancer. One major hurdle Wilt and his colleagues faced was that they couldn't discern what different research groups "meant" when they described erectile dysfunction—or, for that matter, urinary or rectal incontinence. Even the doctors doing research and caring for patients could not agree on a uniform definition of these conditions.

Steven Baum reflected on his reactions to the two surgeons. The first surgeon reinforced the side of Steven that wanted to believe, and the second one amplified his sense of doubt.

Steven understood that he was in a "hot" frame of mind when he saw the first surgeon. Frightened and anxious, he was ready to sign on immediately, as was his wife, to surgery. But by the time he'd arrived for his second opinion after reading and talking to others, he was "cool" and better able to absorb information. Steven reflected, "My goal as a psychologist is to help people accept the uncertainty of life. You take on reality, you pull the curtain back and see that there is no wizard, and that you have to decide for yourself. But still I was attracted to the first urologist because his approach is so paternal, in a way it frees me from worry. I didn't like the uncertainty that comes with the second urologist's telling me I have a 50 percent chance of incontinence and impotence. I needed to explore other options."

Steven then investigated radiation therapy, although he knew that the size of his gland made this approach less than optimal. The radiation therapist explained that first he could be treated with hormonal therapy that might reduce the size of the gland, and then he would potentially receive radiation. This approach seemed even more uncertain to him.

Steven then consulted a medical oncologist expert in prostate cancer. This doctor made the case for "watchful waiting." "You have at least a 50 percent chance of the prostate cancer not killing you if you do nothing," the medical oncologist told Baum. "And if you die of something else twenty years from now, never having suffered from the cancer, then I win and cancer loses, even though I didn't do anything. This is a real option for you." This plan appealed to Steven. Maybe he could get by without any treatment at all.

When we spoke with Steven, he said, "I feel like I'm at a crossroads with about four or five different paths in front of me." His primary care doctor told him, "The hard thing is you are going to have lots of options and there is really not a clear best option." Steven was familiar with the work of the psychologists Barry Schwartz and Sheena Iyengar, who have written extensively about the paradox of choice. Contrary to conventional thinking, having many options can be more distressing than having fewer options and can impede our ability to make a sound decision, or even any decision. Fewer choices can lessen the cognitive burden that comes with having to examine many options. But the wrong choice can lead not only to disappointment, but also to regret.

In his own practice, Steven Baum had listened to countless patients articulate their deep regret about events in their lives—a divorce that could have been avoided, a rift with family or a friend that might have been repaired, an investment chosen unwisely. Steven was determined to do his best to avoid regret. He told us that "I follow the same process in making every decision in my life, whether it's to buy a certain car, sell my apartment, get married, or have a child. I get all the information and then sit with myself and think. Here," he continued, "I need to know that I have seen into my own head and the heads of my doctors—my own feelings and their feelings. At some point, I ask myself, What can I live with? Which choice would be the one that I couldn't live with, and which one would be the choice I could live with? And then I know that I've gone through my process and have achieved a clear understanding.

"What happens in the beginning is that I'm not sure, and I'm running all these different scenarios through my mind. And then I reach a point where I start to see what's right and what's wrong for me. It's a deliberative process, and each person's process is different based on who they are and their history. Somebody else clearly would want to have surgery right away, and that might be right for them, and I may end up there as well, but I'm not there yet. I have to answer the voice in my head that says, 'You know, if you were smart enough or good enough or enough of a man, you would just make your choice now.' But I have come to believe, having made mistakes by being impulsive, that for me decisions of this kind should not be made quickly. Dithering and obsessing and trawling over not only the information but the feelings is what I need to do."

Several months later, still undecided, Steven Baum ran into an old friend at a coffee shop in Westwood. In short order, the conversation turned to Steven's dilemma about choosing a treatment and a doctor. His friend suggested that he speak with Andy Goodman, a lawyer in West Los Angeles, who had just been through treatment for prostate cancer. As it happened, Baum and Goodman had crossed paths years before when their children were in school together. "It seemed *bashert*," Steven told us, using the Yiddish word for "fated." "I got together with Andy, and he told me about the surgeon who had operated on him. But we also talked about sex, in a really honest way. It was like being in college, but this time you were saying it as it really was, no posturing, no exaggerating performance." Andy Goodman detailed how his sex life had been with his wife before his prostate cancer and what they were doing now to try to reclaim gratifying relations.

Steven realized that he had found a person who closely resembled him in terms of background, culture, and mind-set. "It's so interesting," Steven observed. "You are dealing with uncertainties, and you have been told what the numbers are, but you can't really understand what the numbers mean for you. Some people keep looking for more numbers, asking more questions about the statistics on incontinence or impotence or some other issue. But people like me rely on narratives. You want to know what the experience was like, both the experience of the treatment and living with its aftermath. It seemed that Andy Goodman was the best source for me. I saw myself in him and, as best it could be, believed I could see my future before me."

Some researchers raise concerns about this kind of approach to making medical decisions. They argue that anecdotes are simply that, the "*n* of 1," single experiences that can distort thinking by their potent impact, creating an availability bias. But Daniel Gilbert of Harvard University, who has published seminal research studies demonstrating how difficult it is to forecast what you will actually experience, found that listening to other people's personal experiences sometimes may be the best way to make these decisions. In a particularly noteworthy article entitled, "The Surprising Power of Neighborly Advice," published in *Science*, Gilbert shows that we are more likely to accurately predict what we will experience in the future by learning of the experiences of other people. The key, of course, is finding similar people. In Gilbert's study, the primary determinant of similarity involved social and demographic aspects, specifically a person's age and shared status as an undergraduate at Harvard College. We would add that all of us may benefit from hearing the stories of people who are similar to us not only in terms of gender, age, and socioeconomic or educational level, but also in mind-set, orientation, cultural background, and temperament. A "kindred spirit" was what Steven Baum was seeking: a man who would serve as a mirror to himself.

A few weeks later, we spoke with Steven again. "I decided I couldn't live with the cancer in me. If it grew out of control and I could have prevented it, I would regret it. I wanted to see my children grow up. I wanted that cancer out. So I eliminated watchful waiting. It had become watchful worrying. And radiation therapy wasn't certain enough. It was going to be surgery." The surgeon who had performed Andy Goodman's operation did the traditional open approach at one of the medical centers in the Los Angeles area. "I wanted that surgeon."

The urologist performed a so-called nerve-sparing operation and believed that he had done the best that could be done to prevent trauma to the nerves and preserve sexual function. "The news was really good," Steven said. "The urologist said that the cancer did not extend to the margins of the prostate gland, and he didn't think anything was left behind. He told me, 'Your prostate is where it should be, in the pathology lab.'" Steven told us, "I feel in a way reborn, meaning that now I will learn to live a new life, drawing on what I've learned in the past, and trying my best to adapt."

Steven Baum is aware of the extraordinary human capacity to

adapt. What we first imagine to be severely limiting can prove to be less destructive to quality of life because we can find alternative sources of gratification. Baum, as a psychologist, said that adaptation is often the goal of his work with his patients. Many of us adapt to frustrating and debilitating situations to a degree that surprises us. People paralyzed by accidents or by degenerative neurological disorders, some two years after losing motor function, often consider themselves to be as happy as they were before their loss. Many patients with a colostomy, a change that is often viewed with dread and despair, eventually reclaim a sense of happiness and satisfaction close to that before their colon was removed. Richard Cohen, who developed multiple sclerosis and colon cancer at a relatively young age, described his own trajectory of adaptation in his memoir, *Blindsided*; he later profiled other people with muscular dystrophy, inflammatory bowel disease, and advanced lymphoma. The capacity for adaptation was stunning in Cohen's personal story and in his profiles of others.

Research studies show that all of us initially overestimate the ultimate impact of illness and its unpleasant side effects because we tend to focus on the negative and neglect the numerous positives in our lives. Daniel Kahneman, the Nobel laureate who did seminal work in cognitive psychology and decision making, emphasizes how this "focusing illusion" distorts our perceptions and plagues efforts to accurately envision the future. We often underestimate the reservoir of our resilience, the fact that we can adapt, and regress, and then strive to adapt again. Over time, we learn to expand those parts of life that still provide gratification and seek fulfillment in venues we had previously overlooked.

After intensive treatment for prostate cancer, Dana Jennings, a *New York Times* editor, wrote eloquently in that newspaper: "Despite everything that has happened the last couple of years, I'm a lucky man.

I love my work, I'm blessed with two fine sons, and I have my compassionate and indispensable wife to snuggle with on these winter nights. Everything else will mend in its own time."

When we checked in with Matt Conlin again six months after his surgery, we found that he had begun to adapt to his side effects. He was focused on his parents' longevity, calculating that with his cancer gone, he would now live a long and healthy life. He decided to cut back on some projects at work so that he and his wife could take a leisurely trip to Paris and a gastronomic tour of France. With his daughter's upcoming wedding, he was already dreaming of grandchildren.

Neither Matt Conlin's nor Steven Baum's story is finished. For some men, the side effects of urinary incontinence and erectile dysfunction lessen over time. But even if these problems persist for Matt and Steven, they will likely adapt.

Six

—————

Autonomy and Coping

On an unseasonably chilly October evening, Julie Brody pulled off her T-shirt to put on a flannel nightgown and get into bed. As she lifted the shirt, her hand grazed a tiny bump under her left arm. "It was extraordinary that I noticed it," Julie later told us. She asked her husband if he could feel it. He thought he could.

"You should go and get it checked out tomorrow," he said.

"It's the kind of thing I would ignore, because I'm very doctor-averse," Julie told us. "But in my jovial manner, I called my gynecologist and said, 'I seem to have this bit of a lump under my arm. It's probably nothing.'"

The doctor responded with clear concern. "I'm booking you for a mammogram today. Hang up the phone and clear your calendar."

Julie Brody, a short, slim, forty-two-year-old woman with a page-boy haircut and tortoiseshell glasses, had built a small, successful art gallery on the West Coast. She had always been healthy, and her only doctor was her gynecologist. She ate organic foods whenever possible, exercised regularly, and made sure she got adequate sleep. "All the women in my family are very strong and healthy," Julie said. Her grandmother had lived to one hundred and five, and her mother, still vigorous as she approached eighty, had never been hospitalized except to give birth.

Despite the stress of running a gallery and dealing with high-strung artists and intense buyers, Julie told us that she was not a "worrier." "I'm almost pathologically positive. 'It's going to be okay' is the mantra in my mind. There was no one with breast cancer in my family. And anyway, I had a normal mammogram two months earlier.

"I had a meeting waiting outside my office, a young up-and-coming artist with his lawyer. I had to tell them the meeting was not happening, and off I went to the radiologist. Right then and there, they found I had not one but two lumps. One of the lumps was in the breast, and the other one was a lymph node. The radiologist told me right in the middle of the hallway that it looked like cancer even before the biopsy. I'm not one who's going to gush tears." Julie paused. "I was like, 'Oh, that's too bad.' But I would feel terrible for the person who would be knocked on the floor by that."

Within a week, a surgeon removed the two lumps, as well as several other lymph nodes under her arm. As expected, the breast lump and one of the lymph nodes proved to be cancerous. It turned out that Julie hadn't felt the cancer in her breast when she had removed her T-shirt; instead, she'd felt the lump in the adjacent lymph node. "The amazing thing, the radiologist said, was that I felt it at all, because it was so small. It was one of those 'believe in fate' kinds of things." The radiologist retrieved her earlier mammograms but found no abnormalities. "So within two months, a lump had grown in my breast, and then shot off to the lymph node."

In contrast with Matt Conlin and Steven Baum, who received repeated reassurance from their doctors, Julie was given clear and urgent messages. "I felt I had to move quickly, to find the 'best of the best.'" She paused. "That's what we call it in my work—everyone is always trying to find the 'best of the best.'" It's "the best new young artist, the best photographer for the catalog, the best lawyer to write up the contracts. And I believe these people really do have qualities that make them better than anyone else. Now, I needed to know who was the best of the best in breast cancer. I discovered a new way to use my Rolodex." She learned that several of her clients sat on the boards of hospitals, and others had raised money for cancer organizations, so she contacted them. "I got their lists of the best cancer specialists in the state. I put together all the lists and saw who was repeated." Quickly, it became clear to Julie that one oncologist was at the top.

Mary Frances Luce, a researcher on decision making at Duke University, points out that trying to find "the best doctor" or "the best hospital" is, in part, a form of coping. Patients with a serious diagnosis cannot avoid the reality that they will have to make many difficult decisions. Looming behind each choice is the possibility of a negative outcome—an effective therapy might have debilitating and lasting side effects, or the disease, even if treated in the most effective way, might not be cured. Choices must be made, one option selected rather than another; none is guaranteed to succeed, and each has risks. Luce and other researchers term this "decisional conflict," and it is a major source of emotional stress for patients already dealing with the physical difficulties of a disease and its treatment.

People try to cope with decisional conflict in different ways. For those with deep religious faith, prayer and a belief in God's benevolence may provide comfort and a sense that "He will guide." Care from "the best," in Luce's formulation, is another coping mechanism, a way to avoid "hot" decision making by dialing down the emotional temperature to a more tolerable level. The patient reassures herself that she can reduce the uncertainty of choosing among difficult options and increase the odds of success at the "best" hospital with the "best" specialist.

The oncologist "at the top of everyone's list," Julie told us, "was the one I wanted." An art collector she knew was a trustee of the doctor's hospital and contacted him on her behalf. The specialist was expecting Julie's call. "I would love to come in and talk to you about my situation and understand what the options are and what you recommend," she said.

"There's really no need for a lot of discussion, I'll know what is best for you. You're going to get great care here." He paused. "I guarantee you're going to love us."

I don't know that I'm going to love you, Julie thought.

"I'm speaking at a cancer conference in Europe this coming week, but I'll see you as soon as I get back next week."

"Can I really wait a week?" she asked.

"I assure you, a week will not be a problem."

Julie told us that "he seemed to be saying he knows what I like and what I need before even sitting down with me or hearing my story, or finding out who I am. It felt like a one-way street—with no input from my end. This really bothered me." Her intuition made her feel that perhaps this was not the right doctor for her. But powerfully pulling on Julie were the opinions of the people on her Rolodex, who viewed this doctor as the "best of the best." It seemed self-defeating to not be under his care. What benefit might he offer that, in the end, could make all the difference? Would not choosing him hurt her chance to be cured?

"It was one of those really difficult pivot points," Julie recalled. She didn't want to decide impulsively. She imagined one day regretting her decision either way—whether she chose him or another oncologist. She was caught between two visions of future regret.

We saw the negative effect of regret with Lisa Norton after her failed foot surgery. This was regret felt in retrospect. Here, Julie Brody was anticipating regret. Her "pathologically positive" attitude had evaporated. Her mantra that "it's going to be okay" had vanished. Instead of the steady calm she felt in tackling problems at work, Julie was gripped by a sense of fear and anxiety, feeling she had to act quickly. Her gynecologist had made her clear her calendar and go right in for the mammogram and biopsy. Her mammogram was normal two months ago, but now she had cancer not only in the breast, but in a lymph node. She felt time was of the essence. In the paradigm of "hot/cold" decision making, she was poised to make a feverish decision. Anticipation of regret helped her to cool down. But Julie still had a decision to make. Should she choose this doctor or look for someone else? She realized that she had to reach out to someone who understood her dilemma, someone she trusted who knew her personally, and someone on the inside, someone with medical knowledge.

Julie called her gynecologist. She listened carefully to Julie's story. "It is true, he's an outstanding oncologist. But there isn't just one 'best' doctor—there are many excellent oncologists who can provide superb care for you."

We are often asked by patients, family, and friends who is "the best" surgeon, "the best" dermatologist, "the best" pediatrician. We respond similarly that there is no one "best doctor." There are many physicians in each field with deep experience, excellent clinical judgment, and strong communication skills.

"Let me suggest another oncologist that I've worked closely with," the gynecologist said. "This is a doctor whose judgment I respect, and several of my patients have worked well with him. I'll help get you an appointment right away, and then you can see the other oncologist when he gets back from his trip."

H ow do people pick their doctors? According to data from the nonprofit Center for Studying Health System Change, in 2007 an estimated twenty-five million adult Americans sought a new primary care doctor, and more than sixty million looked for a new specialist. Of those adults who found a new primary care physician, fully half relied on recommendations from friends and relatives, and more than a third also drew on recommendations from doctors, nurses, and other medical personnel. When searching for a specialist, the most frequent referral came from the patient's primary care physician, in almost seven in ten instances. One in five patients used recommendations from friends and relatives. In seeking either a new primary care physician or a specialist, only a small fraction relied on information from the Internet, magazines, or other media; such information is of two types, subjective and quantitative. Subjective information includes patients' personal narratives and testimonials about their experiences with specific physicians. For some people seeking a physician, these sources effectively extend their circle of family and friends and influence their choice of doctor. Quantitative information is presented by insurers, government agencies, and nonprofit and for-profit organizations. It's very appealing to imagine that you could reliably choose the right doctor using numerical data.

Indeed, health policy planners and insurance companies increasingly promote the idea that patients should choose their doctors based on report cards that provide metrics on "quality of care." We live in a culture where metrics are increasingly touted as essential in evaluating performance. To be sure, there are certain numbers a patient should know. For example, every surgeon follows a learning curve with a particular operation or instrument or technology. The numbers of procedures performed gives a rough idea of how skillfully the surgeon uses these techniques. And information on safety, like the percentage of postoperative infections at a given hospital, is meaningful. Yet the metrics used in rating doctors fail to measure the key attribute of clinical judgment, how a doctor molds care to the individual patient. Rather, the metrics are based largely on lowest-common-denominator care, like whether a doctor regularly checks a patient's blood sugar level or blood pressure, and also include measures of cost and efficiency. Furthermore, a doctor who avoids patients with multiple medical problems, such as diabetes with kidney failure and heart disease, will have better "outcomes" because he's cherry-picking healthier patients, leaving the sickest ones to others. We find the famous statement attributed to Albert Einstein apt: "Not everything that can be counted counts, and not everything that counts can be counted."

Insurers are also developing report cards on so-called higher-cost and lower-cost doctors, assessing the costs of care associated with a particular physician. A recent article in the *New England Journal of Medicine* showed that these statistics are often unreliable. The same physician can be rated as high-cost on one report card and low-cost on another.

Such limitations have not stopped insurance companies from launching advertising campaigns promising that if you use their metrics and report cards, you will get the right doctor and have the right outcome. This promise cannot be kept.

In one ad, an attractive, athletic woman is running in a sunny park against a background of digits. Across her midsection reads the tagline: KNOWLEDGE IN NUMBERS STRENGTH IN NUMBERS HUMANITY IN NUMBERS COMFORT IN NUMBERS HEALTH IN NUMBERS.[SM] The message below the image: "STRENGTH: You have a tricky medical condition. You need to make a medical decision. You would like to know you are choosing the right doctor, choosing the right procedure, and will have the right outcome. It's only human to feel this way."

As this ad shows, insurance companies understand decisional conflict, the patient's "only human" fears and anxiety about choosing the "right" doctor and choosing the "right" treatment. The insurers want you to believe that the most agonizing truth of medical care—its uncertainty—is no longer a concern. These companies claim that they can resolve decisional conflict: If you rely on their numbers, you will get the right outcome. But no one can guarantee that you will get the right outcome. The FDA exercises oversight on truth in drug advertising, and we believe the same should be done for claims by insurers about outcomes.

Julie went to see the oncologist her gynecologist suggested. "It felt like he had all the time in the world to talk to me. And he seemed to be focused on me as an individual. But he made it clear there are always risks and uncertainties in cancer treatment." That made her anxious. Maybe she should choose the doctor who was the "best of the best." "I really had to think about which oncologist to choose. But finally I realized there would still be risks even with the best of the best." She decided she would begin her treatment with the second specialist. "It was a difficult decision. But it really helped that a doctor I knew and trusted validated that this oncologist was a good choice.

"Dr. Best of the Best—when I called and told him that I'd be seeing this other oncologist—replied, 'Of course, I'm great, he's great. Whatever.'"

Almost immediately after choosing her oncologist, Julie Brody was faced with a difficult decision. After her lumpectomy, the surgeon told her that she would be getting chemotherapy and that she wouldn't need radiation. But the oncologist she had chosen disagreed; he felt that radiation would reduce the risk that the cancer would return. They told her the final decision would be hers. This is the type of "decisional conflict" that Duke's Mary Frances Luce highlights as a major source of stress for patients.

"My oncologist gave me strong advice," Julie told us. "But he didn't dictate. Not only did he explain the benefits of radiation with regard to treatment of the cancer, but also how radiation has downsides, increasing the risk of long-term complications, like other malignancies, and how it changes the tissue that is radiated, making reconstructive surgery after a mastectomy more challenging."

Julie said it was a lot to absorb, and she had to think about the conflicting opinions. A few days after the appointment, the oncologist called Julie on her cell phone. She walked into her office behind the gallery, a quiet place where she could speak privately. "He told me that he had presented my case to a clinical conference at the hospital," Julie said. "There were other oncologists, as well as my surgeon and other surgeons, and radiation specialists."

The oncologist told her that during the discussion of her case, "there were some people who thought I didn't need radiation, and some who did." Her oncologist once again reviewed the pros and cons of the treatment. "And then he said, 'I just didn't hear anything that convinced me that you do not need radiation. But in the end, this is your decision—I will support you either way.'"

That made a deep impression on Julie. "He definitely had to talk me through it four or five times. It wasn't as though he presented his point of view to me and I said, 'Okay! Great, radiate me.'

"My doctor was saying, 'Here, you can look behind the curtain. You can see.' It's not like he said there are no other points of view. For some people, telling them might have resulted in doubt about his ability or lack of confidence in his judgment. I felt that he was showing me everything. But I still had to make the choice."

Mary Frances Luce found that some patients seek to mitigate the "emotional costs" of making difficult decisions by directly and repeatedly "attacking" the complexity of the choices they face. Luce terms this "vigilant decision making." Matt Conlin embodied this approach. Constantly crunching the numbers, contacting more than twenty different doctors, trying to delve deeply into research studies culled from Internet searches, Matt was trying to reduce decisional conflict by finding small but significant differences that would tip the scales toward one treatment or another. But for many patients this is simply too difficult, both technically and emotionally. They believe they don't have the capacity to critically assess the vast sea of conflicting information.

Julie didn't feel confident to interpret what she found on the Internet. "I'm not going to become a doctor, like some certified specialist, in a few months. So finding that right doctor was so important." She decided to undergo radiation treatment. "I know a lot of people who had cancer, and either have doctors whom they don't trust, or don't like, or who themselves believe in their own power of research. So they do a lot of scoping out on the Internet and find all sorts of studies. But how do you really know what all those numbers mean?"

Depending on another person as her primary guide in decision making was alien to Julie. She was used to being the boss, overseeing all the choices made in her gallery—which artists to represent, when to schedule an opening, and which guests to invite. She listened to advice, would at times question her own thinking, but ultimately held sway over every decision. She was used to being in charge, functioning with a high level of autonomy.

Autonomy is a primary right of all patients, and it is widely assumed that patients always want a major role in directing their medical treatment and care. But studies indicate that there is considerable diversity in how much control patients want to have. One report of more than one thousand Canadian women with breast cancer showed that 22 percent wanted to select their own cancer treatment, 44 percent wanted to select treatment together with their doctor, and 34 percent wanted to delegate completely the choice to their physician. Interestingly, over the course of their care, less than half believed that they had achieved their desired level of control in decision making.

At the pivot point of considering radiation therapy, Julie felt she had reached a sufficient level of trust and confidence in her oncologist that she could cede control to him. This didn't mean that he shielded her from the complexities of her choices or presented his opinion as infallible. He didn't pretend, as she put it, "to be an oracle." Julie still wanted to know where she was going and how she would get there, but her doctor was the pilot, because he not only had the technical knowledge needed to navigate, but, she believed, had gained a sense of her as an individual and would factor in her values and goals at each point along the way. Here, Julie welcomed her doctor offering his preferences, because he did so in a transparent and considered way. This is in contrast with what we saw earlier in the case of Patrick Baptiste, where his physician projected his own treatment preference onto Patrick without first assessing how much input and control Patrick wanted.

Julie told us, "My oncologist really believed that it would be better for me to do the radiation, and this is where, I think, you have to believe your doctor is trying to do the absolute best for you. That's the point of seeking the right doctor.

"It was lucky for me," Julie told us, "that I was able to put my faith in my doctor."

For Julie, ceding some autonomy to him made such a miserable period in her life more bearable. "I know somebody who had cancer at the same time that I did. She had a completely different experience. She didn't trust her doctor, and that gave her a lot of anxiety and uncertainty—sleepless nights online, a lot of e-mailing around. Her outcome was good, which is wonderful, but . . ." Julie paused. "But, it was like a constant struggle. The burden was so much greater."

After she agreed to undergo radiation therapy, Julie felt that everything was settled, that her treatment plan was clearly defined. But then she received test results showing that she had a mutation in a BRCA gene. Her oncologist had previously explained that the BRCA1 and BRCA2 genes are normally involved in limiting damage to DNA, so when either is mutated, damaged DNA can more readily change a cell from normal to cancerous. Mutated BRCA genes are particularly common among women of Eastern European Jewish heritage, like Julie, but they are also found in other ethnic and racial groups. In most cases, the mutation is inherited from a parent—but not always. Her oncologist had also told her that mutated BRCA genes markedly increase the likelihood of developing breast cancer in any remaining breast tissue. Furthermore, the mutation increases the risk of ovarian cancer.

Julie told us, "I believe you should know everything about your condition. The more that is known, the better the doctor can treat you." Now, she faced a new set of choices. She recalled how her oncologist "laid out all the options." They spoke for more than an hour.

He told her the most proven way for a woman with a BRCA mutation to prevent future cancer is to have both breasts removed, a double mastectomy, and also have the ovaries taken out. "This reduces the risk of breast and ovarian cancer by more than 90 percent," he said.

Julie paused, and her voice became heavy. "I'll tell you," she said, "I didn't like the idea of mastectomy, particularly a double mastectomy."

Julie asked him, "What if I don't want that surgery?" He explained that another option was to take a medication like tamoxifen, which has been shown in some studies to decrease the risk of future breast cancer by as much as 50 percent. "But we really don't know if that is true for women like you with BRCA mutations. And the medication does not prevent ovarian cancer." He further explained that if Julie did not want surgery, she would be closely monitored for breast cancer with mammograms and MRI scans. But this kind of monitoring has not been proven to be as reliable as a mastectomy in saving lives. With respect to monitoring for ovarian cancer, he explained, "ultrasound and blood tests don't reliably detect ovarian cancer at an early stage."

Julie left the appointment without reaching a decision. "It was an awful lot to absorb," she told us. "He didn't press me to choose, and emphasized how personal the choice is for each woman." Julie's earlier preference to cede decision making to her doctor shifted. Here, she wanted to clearly assert her preferences. She thought about the statistics that had been given to her. Then she went on the Internet. After looking at several decision aids, she realized that she would not base her choice strictly on numbers. "I didn't want to have any sense that I hadn't done everything I could do. My breasts, even though they're small, I knew I'd miss them. But in the end, I did everything: I chose the double mastectomy, had my ovaries removed, got chemotherapy and radiation therapy. And I came out feeling that if this cancer comes back, there was nothing that I skipped that could have prevented it."

Mary Frances Luce has studied how patients manage the complexity of the choices they face. Some focus on only one aspect of the choice, disregarding the other outcomes. This reduces cognitive effort, lessens decisional conflict, and helps them cope. For example, some people may ignore all the possible side effects of surgery, "shielding themselves," as Luce puts it, from thinking about the pain involved or the risk of being disfigured or debilitated; they focus only on the chance of survival. Others may focus on every potential side effect of surgery, and this detailed deliberation helps them cope. They feel more in control by having weighed each possible outcome, analyzing all aspects of the choice.

Julie told us, "I didn't want to look back and say that I didn't do all I could do." She was again anticipating regret, regret that she might have been able to prevent the one outcome she feared more than anything else, not living to see her children grow up. This led her to reduce the cognitive effort in deciding to undergo surgery. "The ovaries required the least thought because I have two children, and someday I'll be in menopause anyway. And I was told that having the ovaries out was actually a really simple operation." She paused. "Well, it probably is. But when I had my ovaries out, I had already had four months of chemo, and three weeks before that I had had a double mastectomy, so at the time I had my ovaries out, my body was pretty shot."

Despite this, Julie told us, "It's sort of funny. After I recovered from the surgery, I went out with my husband and saw *The Wizard of Oz* on the big screen. And there was a very humorous scene when Dorothy is going down the yellow brick road. This is when she meets the Scarecrow. She is on the yellow brick road and there were something like five yellow brick roads. Which yellow brick road is she supposed to take?"

Julie felt relieved that "I never got to that point, I never felt like there were five yellow brick roads." She was able to lessen her decisional conflict by doing everything that might help improve the chance for cure, despite the impact on her body. Like Steven Baum, she felt that she had gone through her process and didn't need to look back.

Julie Brody is like many other women who are first diagnosed with breast cancer and later discover they carry a BRCA mutation. In one study, 52 percent of such women chose a bilateral or "double" mastectomy after learning that they carried the mutated gene. But what about women who have the BRCA mutation but don't have cancer?

Sara Rosen, a thirty-eight-year-old pastry chef also living on the West Coast, had several aunts and cousins with breast cancer. She agonized for many years before deciding to be tested for the BRCA mutation. "I wasn't sure what I would do with the information," she told us. And she was concerned about the burden it might put on her two teenage daughters. But after Sara's younger sister was diagnosed with breast cancer and was found to be positive for a BRCA1 mutation, she spoke to a genetic counselor and then decided to be tested. Sara's test was positive, and she learned that the likelihood that she would develop breast cancer in the future was between 55 and 85 percent. Her risk for ovarian cancer was 36 to 63 percent. Sara consulted with several oncologists and read about her options on the Internet. Her mammogram, MRI scan, CA-125 blood test for ovarian cancer, and pelvic ultrasound were all normal. Since she wasn't planning to have more children, she decided to have her ovaries removed. But Sara declined breast surgery, choosing to take tamoxifen instead.

About half of women who carry a BRCA mutation with a normal pelvic ultrasound and blood tests are like Sara Rosen and choose to have their ovaries removed. But Sara is like the vast majority of women with BRCA who do not have a diagnosis of breast cancer—they don't choose mastectomy. In one study, only 3 percent of such women chose bilateral mastectomy within the first year of learning that they carried a BRCA mutation.

A drastic intervention like removing both breasts and both ovaries to prevent a disease you don't have and may never get presents the extreme of decisional conflict and loss aversion. The losses are many and profound. A woman faces major surgery, with the attendant risks of pain, disfigurement, scarring, infection, and bleeding. Further, losing her breasts and ovaries challenges a woman's self-image. The immediate onset of menopausal symptoms after their ovaries are removed makes many women feel miserable, with hot flashes that disrupt sleep, exhaustion, mood swings, depression, and impaired sexual function. Although many women adapt over time, the adaptation process may be lengthy and incomplete. These were the thoughts in Sara's mind.

Two years later, Sara's younger sister died of metastatic breast cancer. "I could not escape the thought that I would be next," Sara told us. "Availability," a dramatic event that deeply influences you, proved a powerful force in changing Sara's thinking and overcoming loss aversion. She decided to undergo bilateral mastectomy. Fortunately, no breast cancer was found. Sara was relieved and told us, "I believe I made the right decision, but it hasn't been easy. Not easy at all."

Everyone knows what I've been through," Julie told us, "and now I can help others." She had shared the details of her illness with numerous friends and all her co-workers. Julie believed that sharing her experiences lightened the burden of her arduous treatment. Now she has found herself on other people's Rolodexes: "I'm getting so many calls for advice." She feels, not surprisingly, that she is "educated" about cancer. "I try to point out to the person who is going through cancer how you can have the best experience." Julie was now focused not on the "best doctor," but on the "best experience."

"Part of the experience is determined by the doctor," she said. "But not only him and his team. There was my support network of friends. All caring people, all who care about me."

What constitutes the "best experience" is highly personal. Angela Balducci, forty-four years old, liked being a stay-at-home mom in her midwestern community. Her two children were now in high school, and Angela's days were filled with shuttling them to various activities. Petite and athletic, she made time to exercise at the yoga studio and on her elliptical trainer. Angela had been an English major in college and remained an avid reader. She kept a stack of novels in her car, devouring them whenever she had some time. While on a trip with her son, a varsity baseball player who was competing at regional play-offs, Angela developed an ache in her upper back. "I thought it was sleeping in cheap hotels and sitting in the car for hours upon hours driving to the games," she recalled. After more than a week without relief from stretching, she went to her primary care physician. The doctor examined her but didn't find anything abnormal. Because Angela had smoked briefly as a teenager, he ordered a chest X-ray. "I also have a little bit of asthma, so he wanted to look at my lungs." Angela paused. The memory still weighed heavily upon her. "He called back two hours later and said that they had found a mass between my lungs. My God, it moved so fast. I found out on a Tuesday, had a CT scan on Wednesday, and a surgeon was called to perform a biopsy. They knew by Thursday that it was Hodgkin's lymphoma," Angela said.

In contrast with Matt Conlin and Steven Baum, who had time to choose their doctors and think about treatment over months, Angela Balducci had a cancer that had to be treated quickly. She recalled feeling "paralyzed." All she could think of was dying, leaving her two growing children and husband without her. She turned to her husband, who became her "eyes and ears" in her interactions with her doctors.

Things moved rapidly. Angela was seen by the oncologist at the community hospital where her primary care physician worked. She outlined the treatment plan for Angela's Hodgkin's lymphoma, and Angela began treatment. But then she and her husband felt she should get a second opinion at a cancer center. Her local oncologist helped her arrange this. Angela and her husband went that same week to speak with a lymphoma specialist at the nearby cancer center.

Angela waited in the clinic, watching a stream of people pass by, many bald and frail, some in wheelchairs. After forty minutes, she was ushered into an examination room. A nurse's aide took her vital signs and then had Angela step on the scale. "Oh, my God," Angela said, "I'm down seven pounds." The aide shrugged silently and put an ID bracelet on Angela's wrist.

"When I was in the waiting room at the cancer center, it felt very depressing," Angela told us. "Those people were much sicker than I was." Soon the lymphoma specialist, a tall, thin, older man who spoke with a British accent, entered. He went over her history, examined her briefly, and then detailed the treatment that she would receive. "He was very professional," Angela told us, "but honestly he looked totally bored. In fact, he said that I was a 'typical case.'"

The doctor suggested the same treatment that the oncologist at her local hospital had. "Everyone offered the same chemotherapy and radiation," she said. Angela had several friends who had been diagnosed with breast cancer, and she reflected on the difference between her case and theirs. "It took them two, three, four weeks to think out what their plan was. At each hospital, different treatments were recommended. I think that's more agonizing."

Angela continued, "Things were moving so fast and were so serious, the doctors had to make decisions for us. I didn't have any real choices. They didn't say A or B or C—which one do you want? On the decision front, for me, with Hodgkin's disease, it was very clear what had to be done. Unless I wanted to be on an experimental protocol, they told me, it was about the same everywhere. It seemed pretty linear."

Successful treatment of Hodgkin's lymphoma is one of the great triumphs of modern oncology. Over the past few decades, researchers in North America and Europe have systematically studied the optimal therapy for different stages and various subtypes of the cancer. These studies have developed and refined to a high degree therapy for Hodgkin's lymphoma. Cure rates are higher than 70 percent for tumors detected in their early stages and more than 50 percent even for late-stage, widespread Hodgkin's lymphoma. There is still some debate among experts about the optimal timing of chemotherapy and radiation and exactly which drugs to use in order to limit long-term damage to the heart and lungs and the risk of a second malignancy like leukemia. While this research continues, patients who don't want to participate in an experimental protocol can be reassured that there is a deep foundation of knowledge upon which to base their treatment.

"Oh, God, I feel so lucky. I mean, the first thing you think when you get cancer is, 'Thank God it's me, not the kids.' And then there are people who don't have a doctor, don't have insurance, and don't have a job. And the bottom line is, Hodgkin's has a high cure rate. But I still had to go through the treatment. And the question was where?"

Angela felt anonymous in the cancer center. She wasn't at all reassured by the comment that she was "typical." Rather, she felt that she was seen as "just another case." What might seem like a small gesture, the nurse's silent shrug when Angela expressed dismay about losing seven pounds, reinforced this sense. When patients feel sick, frightened, and vulnerable, seemingly innocuous statements and actions can have tremendous impact. Angela's experience that day clinched her decision to be treated at her community hospital. Other people have the opposite experience and find that a large, bustling cancer center gives them a needed sense of confidence.

Yet Angela still wondered if the oncologist in her community hospital was the right doctor for her. She wanted reassurance, and, like Julie Brody, she found it from a medical professional she knew and trusted. A friend of Angela's was a nurse at the community hospital. "I called her right away. She'd been working there for twenty years. I gave her the name of the doctor that I had seen in oncology. She gave me the rundown on her." The nurse knew the doctor Angela was asking about and told her that she'd been trained at the cancer center and that she was highly competent and very compassionate. Angela appreciated her friend's words, then confided that she was dreading reading about Hodgkin's on the Internet. "The nurse told me 'You don't have to look on the Internet if you don't want to. It can get really scary. Often what you read about online is not the mainstream case. It's not always reliable. It can be just more information to flip out over.'"

Angela felt comforted by her conversation with this nurse. "It was a tremendous relief to feel that I was in good hands. And also a great relief not to feel I needed to hear every person's story about Hodgkin's disease.

"In the beginning," she said, "I put everything on my husband. For the first month, I just sort of sat in the corner and cried, so he was the one who was taking down all the information—what the drug protocol was going to be, managing all of the medications I had to take at home, scheduling family things."

Angela restricted knowledge of her condition to a few close confidantes. She didn't want every conversation to center on her illness and treatment. Many people seek out other cancer patients or survivors for information or advice, but Angela didn't. When she was offered the opportunity to join a support group, she declined and explained, "The only help I want is someone lying on the table for me. That's what I want. If you want to help me, that's what you can do. Otherwise leave me alone."

Angela largely kept her diagnosis a secret, following the principle of "need to know." Although she had physician friends, she kept her situation private even from them. She worried that some people would drain her energy by engaging her in discussions about her disease, asking probing questions about her feelings and her fears. Uninvited suggestions from well-meaning friends, about someone they knew with Hodgkin's lymphoma or someone with a different kind of lymphoma who they thought had seen a different doctor or received another treatment, would do nothing but raise decisional conflict for Angela. She told us she had no emotional reserve for such people who, with the best intentions, might end up getting more from her than they would give her. "I estimated 98 percent of the people would turn out to be better than you ever thought they were, and 2 percent just want to live off your bad news."

Angela wasn't the only person we met who kept her diagnosis mostly to herself. And there can be many reasons why patients might not want to share their medical information. A thirty-two-year-old university professor who had chronic leukemia wanted to avoid having her disease become the focus of every conversation she had, but she also worried that she wouldn't get tenure, that her condition might affect her status at work. "My promotion could be on the line," she said, so "only my family and my closest friend knew." It isn't just cancer that people may be reluctant to share. A retired construction worker developed cardiomyopathy, a weakness of the heart muscle.

The cause of his heart failure was not identified, and its future course was uncertain. He told his wife but didn't want his grown children to know. "Their worries would only make me feel worse," he told us.

For Angela, keeping her diagnosis private helped her to preserve her sense of normalcy. She didn't want her disease to subsume her identity. She could talk with friends about her son's baseball games and her daughter's role in the school play without discussing her health. She needed to feel that she was a person, not only a patient, that cancer hadn't changed her entire life. These protective barriers helped her cope. "You have to take everything as it comes," Angela said. "You can't let it consume you."

She also found deep comfort in her oncologist's attention to the personal aspects of her life. "She was always thinking of something that would be better for me," she said. "Often, she went ahead and made phone calls and changed the schedule so I didn't have to miss my son's baseball games. She would just take that extra step. I felt like she cared for me as a person, not just a case that she was managing among many."

The oncologist also told Angela that she often consulted with colleagues to "get a second opinion to check herself." Angela liked that. "I'm more scared of the person who thinks they know everything."

Like Julie Brody, Angela didn't try to become an expert about her disease. "You have to trust people. Teachers teach, and that's how they spend their careers. People like doctors and nurses spend their lives figuring out how to take care of patients."

Carl Schneider points out in his book *The Practice of Autonomy* how in some cases our culture seems to go to extremes, stigmatizing people who don't want to assert control at every step of their illness. We agree with Schneider. In our view, true autonomy means that the patient can decide the limits of his or her autonomy. Further, part of autonomy is defining one's personal way of coping.

We spoke with Angela four months after her treatment ended. There was no sign of Hodgkin's lymphoma, and it's very likely she is cured. Although she hadn't yet gained back all of her weight and strength, she told us that she has returned to her yoga classes. "My oncologist told me that they like to treat lymphoma because it makes them look so good; they bring people back to life. I am getting back to being the person I was."

Seven

Decision Analysis
Meets Reality

P aul Peterson looked again at the spreadsheet on his computer screen. After each blood test, he always entered his results. The data set he had called up displayed his total number of white blood cells. His count was consistently low, between 2,000 and 3,000. Paul understood why: This was a side effect of the medications he took for a muscle disease called polymyositis. These drugs were known to lower white blood cell counts.

He tapped on the keyboard, and a graph appeared, showing what he had already noted on the spreadsheet, that his usually low white blood cell count had risen into the normal range. Something had changed. This bothered him.

Paul sat back in his chair, deep in thought. In his world, everything had to have a rational explanation. He could think of no explanation for the increase in his white count. He was taking the same doses of his medications as always. He took an inventory of his body:

He did not feel sick; he didn't have pain in his muscles or anywhere else, for that matter; his energy level was good; he hadn't had any fevers or sweats to suggest an infection that might raise his white blood count. Nothing seemed off. He never ignored discrepant data, never dismissed as an "outlier" some finding that he couldn't readily understand. There must be a reason his white count had increased.

Paul Peterson grew up on a farm in Kansas and studied engineering in college. After graduation, he took a job in Wichita in a chemical factory, and although he excelled at his work, he soon grew restless. "I wanted to be my own boss," Paul told us. "And that meant pursuing a career where I would be the one laying out the strategy." He returned to school and studied a wide variety of subjects, including anthropology, psychology, sociology, mathematics, and finance, and ultimately obtained a PhD in the field of organizational behavior. Although his faculty adviser suggested he continue on an academic path and ultimately become a professor, Paul's determination to be independent led him in a different direction. He founded a consulting company and advised corporations in the United States and abroad. "My background was key. I applied the principles of rational decision making to show managers how to create the kind of future that met their goals."

Drawing on his mathematical and computer skills, Paul excelled at creating so-called decision trees, analyzing each potential choice a client faced and charting its chances of success or failure. "There literally were thousands of decisions that could be made over a long time frame. I showed the CEO how to get his arms around a very complex series of decisions, where to place resources, what kind of technology was required, what was the optimal management system to put over it. My work was both quantitative and qualitative, and involved making sure that the thought processes brought to bear were rigorous and identified with precision the kinds of risks that were to be taken and the expected benefits that would be reaped."

Now in his fifties, Paul Peterson is a tall, lean man with a full head of red hair. Before his muscle disease, he was a cyclist and lifted weights. His home in Connecticut bordered a forest, and he chopped his own firewood for a wood-burning stove, about eight cords a year. "I was in very good shape," he told us. "Then in the summer of 2000, completely out of the blue, I lost weight, felt weak, had difficulty pushing hills on the bike. I'd never been sick before, so I just kept saying, 'Well, it's probably just stress, my recent divorce, the traveling with my job, no wonder I feel tired, no wonder I feel weak.' It was an awful time. But finally, after almost a year, I went to see my doctor." Over the course of the next year, Paul saw numerous specialists and had blood tests, X-rays, and CT scans. Despite the extensive evaluation, no one was able to make a diagnosis. "Finally, one of the doctors figured it out with a simple blood test, a CPK," Paul said. "I had polymyositis." Polymyositis is a disorder in which the immune system attacks the muscles, causing inflammation with the release of a protein called creatine phosphokinase, CPK. After two years of therapy with potent medications that suppressed the body's immune reaction against his muscles, Paul improved.

The experience of this illness had a profound effect on him. "Here I saw doctors repeatedly failing to come up with my diagnosis. It turned out that it needed just a simple blood test. I passed by a lot of prominent specialists who didn't see that." While Paul had a good relationship with his primary care physician, he had scant trust or confidence in the medical establishment at large. "As a believer in rationality, in decision science, I would say I am a skeptic. A good Socratic skeptic."

Paul tapped the keyboard again, printing out the spreadsheet and graph, and arranged an appointment with the rheumatologist who was overseeing his treatment.

"I don't make much of it," the rheumatologist said, looking at the graph showing the recent rise in white blood count.

"But it's two standard deviations above my usual mean," Paul replied. "I realize it's in the normal range, but that doesn't seem to be normal for me."

The physician examined him, but found nothing worrisome and then sent a repeat set of blood tests. The next morning, Paul heard that his white blood count was again normal, even slightly higher than the previous count. "I'm not concerned," the rheumatologist said. "This is probably just a viral infection that bumped your white count up a bit."

"I was clearly more worried about this than my doctor," Paul told us. "I really pushed at that point to see a specialist, a hematologist. I mean, after having been sick so long with polymyositis, I didn't want unknown things happening."

The hematologist examined Paul and found nothing abnormal. Then he drew a blood sample and smeared a drop onto a glass slide. He studied it himself under the microscope and gave Paul a rational explanation for the changes in his blood counts.

"He told me I had chronic lymphocytic leukemia," Paul said. "That I likely developed it because of my immune condition, and that taking those cytotoxic drugs, even in low doses, caused mutations in my blood cells. So after all those years of treatment, sometimes you come to understand the consequences of previous decisions."

"Chronic lymphocytic leukemia is often a very indolent condition, not like other leukemias," the hematologist explained to Paul. "It can be stable for many, many years without harming you. At this level of white count, and without any sign that it's causing problems, I recommend that we watch you without any treatment."

Paul listened but did not feel particularly reassured. "I'm a Buddhist. I am interested in Eastern ways of thinking, and I'm drawn to Eastern medicine. But here I decided that if this problem was going to be solved, it would be solved by Western medicine. Perhaps I'd modify that approach, complement it with alternative medicine if I needed to, but that would come later."

As soon as he returned home from the appointment, he went on the Internet. He attacked the problem the same way he did in his work as a strategic planner. He tried to define each dimension of the disease—its cause, manifestations, degree of variability, therapies—and then worked to understand the multiple possible outcomes.

In Mary Frances Luce's terminology, Paul Peterson represents the extreme of "vigilant decision making." He was undeterred by the fact that he didn't have a formal education in medicine. "I was educated through the experience of my polymyositis," he told us. "Furthermore, I'm a scientist. I understand how research is conducted, what statistics show and don't show. I was well aware of all the garbage that's out there on the Internet. So I decided to go with top-tier journals, well-accredited papers, authored by specialists who are at recognized institutions."

Paul found that one of the richest sources of research information was from the American Society of Hematology, the professional organization of clinicians and laboratory scientists who study blood diseases like chronic lymphocytic leukemia, also known as CLL. He went through scores of clinical trials, studied numerous protocols, assessed how many patients had been treated in each research report. In some instances, he recalculated the statistics from studies himself using different methodologies. "Often the sample size was relatively small, so you couldn't really draw conclusions, even though the paper had statistics that claimed to be meaningful. I took those studies with a grain of salt."

Like Julie Brody, who used her Rolodex of contacts to find the "best doctor," Paul Peterson created his list of the "best" experts in CLL. He drew on the rosters of faculty at major cancer centers, then culled the list based on their authorship of articles in prominent medical journals. Paul identified three major cancer centers with experts in his type of leukemia who had published a substantial number of articles in recognized medical journals. Some of the best articles, he concluded, came from a major cancer center in the South. "What I really liked was that they compared the treatment protocols and outcomes of a number of different studies, taking a comprehensive approach, critically analyzing the pros and cons of the various therapeutic strategies."

Paul Peterson is in that minority of patients, based on the 2007 survey, who selected a specialist based on information from the Internet. As it happened, his hematologist in Connecticut knew the expert in CLL at that cancer center. "This personal connection between them kind of added to my decision to get a second opinion there," Paul said. As with Julie Brody, the personal endorsement from another doctor carried weight.

The next week, he traveled south to the cancer center. "It's this huge complex," he said. "You see cranes everywhere, and they must have a hundred thousand employees in the facility. I had this gut reaction that it felt like a center of knowledge and expertise." But in his work as a strategic consultant implementing rational decision analysis, Paul had long ago learned to be wary of "gut reactions." He continued, "I was impressed with the management, the way the schedule was already prepared for me. My three days were all set out by time, each appointment and test moving into the next. There was just this incredible efficiency, a sense that everything was well organized, ran smoothly. I said to myself, Okay, these people seem to know how to run patients through here. On the other hand," Paul told us, "it was very large, and that turned me off a bit. There were literally thousands of cancer patients moving through the center at any one time. Also you are walking through the corridors, seeing these people who are incredibly sick, and it's not exactly an up experience."

Paul went to wait in the phlebotomy suite for his blood to be drawn.

"Hey, darling—you, over there," a plump, older woman in a white coat called out with a deep southern drawl. "Yes, you, Red. Come right here, darling, and sit down with me, and we'll get this blood test done."

Paul told us, "It's just a simple experience like that—this woman was so nice to me, made me feel like an individual." This mirrored what Julie Brody observed about her oncologist's office and contributed to what she called "the best experience." Paul elaborated, "It wasn't just, Put your arm down, bam, bam, bam, draw your blood, and out you go. Little things like that made me feel that there was something special about the organization. Not that I was convinced everyone in the hospital would be like that. But it was a nice appetizer to go with the main dish, the hospital."

The next day, Paul saw the doctor. This was the specialist in CLL who had published numerous reports of her own clinical trials and a critique of the field. She was middle-aged, dressed in a starched white coat, with a tall stack of papers on her desk. "I liked her style," Paul told us. "All business."

"I have all of your laboratory studies in front of me," the doctor said. "Let me cut to the chase—it doesn't look good."

Paul was taken aback. "What does that mean, precisely?"

The doctor explained that an analysis of Paul's abnormal white blood cells showed several markers indicating a poor prognosis. His CLL was likely to transform from its current indolent state into an aggressive and potentially lethal disorder.

Paul pressed the hematologist to translate her words into numbers: how likely, over what time frame? What are the trajectories based on a patient's age, gender, time since initial diagnosis, and any other possibly relevant variables? And how good are the data? Paul told us that the specialist didn't answer most of these questions precisely and closed the conversation by saying there was nothing to be done immediately except to monitor his white blood cell count even more closely. The specialist would work in conjunction with Paul's local hematologist in Connecticut.

"I expected it would just be an informational visit," Paul told us. "But it turned out to be much more than that."

Paul was determined to maintain control over his care. He went back and read scientific papers about the kinds of genetic changes that occur in chronic leukemic cells that cause them to multiply rapidly and invade vital organs like the liver and kidneys, wreaking havoc with normal body functions. He went regularly to have his blood count checked and kept close watch on the results. As predicted, his white blood count rose from 10,000 to 20,000 and then reached 30,000. "The hematologist reassured me. He didn't seem at all worried. And I felt fine," Paul recalled. His reading on the Internet confirmed that these white blood cell counts are not routinely treated, since they do no harm. Some seven months later, sitting with the doctor, Paul learned that his total white blood cell count was now just above 50,000.

"We should begin treatment this week," the hematologist said.

Paul told us that "I just walked in for a visit, expecting that we were just watching my blood count, waiting. No one had given me any sign that once it topped a particular number that we somehow passed the threshold. That threshold was in my doctor's mind; I didn't know it existed. I was totally unprepared to hear this. I had recently remarried, and I was planning a vacation with my wife." Paul said he was "completely surprised. And this was just the first of a long series of surprises."

Paul asked the hematologist, "Why exactly now? What were the criteria that necessitated treatment?" He was seeking a clear and cogent rationale based on data.

"My sense is once your count doubles this quickly and goes north of 45,000," the hematologist replied, "it's best to begin."

Paul bristled at the inexact nature of the response. "I felt like it was presented as if I had no choice. Of course, I could have declined chemotherapy. But then what? It was, 'This is what you do, and by the way we are starting in three days.' It really bothered me that the decision rules they were using weren't apparent to me. That's a better way to put it. They had made decisions when I didn't even know the decision was coming. And that was that. I didn't like it. I'm a person who spent his life studying decision making. I would like some warning, telling me, 'We are approaching a place where I'm thinking that we may have to begin treatment,' rather than, 'You have three days and you are into chemotherapy.' Because you don't know what that's going to mean. I read all the horror stories, blogs about side effects, how you lose your hair, you're going to be nauseated, and you can bleed. It hit me like a ton of bricks."

He knew from his research on the Internet that cancer centers often differed from one another in the protocols they favored. Until this point, Paul had felt in control, with a clear understanding of the plan—observation without treatment. Now the ground had shifted suddenly beneath him, and he couldn't get his footing. The hematologist explained that he would be using the protocol recommended by the cancer center where Paul had been evaluated. The doctor gave him information sheets for each drug that he would be taking. "I knew this protocol was the gold standard; I had read about it." Paul's sense of control returned.

He received several cycles of treatment, and for some six months, his leukemia was contained. But then, as predicted, his disease took a more aggressive form, unresponsive to a series of chemotherapy regimens. The specialist at the cancer center proposed that Paul undergo a bone marrow transplant. Here, a donor whose marrow was genetically compatible with Paul's would be found, hopefully a family member. The stem cells from that donor would be infused into Paul and would migrate into his bone marrow after it had been cleared of cancerous cells by high-dose chemotherapy and radiation. In essence, this is a medical resurrection, treating the patient with lethal doses of drugs and then rescuing him with the primitive stem cells that will grow and develop into all of the blood components.

"The doctors present the transplant to you as though it is a decision," Paul said. "Well, I think it's really a pseudodecision. When they asked if I wanted to have a bone marrow transplant, I answered, 'What else is there?' They said, 'Well, you have to have it,' so then the decision was like, 'Well, is it a transplant or is it death?' There was no spectrum of options, no real decision trees. It was transplant or die."

Paul traveled again to the cancer center. He was admitted to the hospital and began the arduous preparation for the transplant. "They make believe that the patient has some level of control," Paul said. "But I think it's an illusion. There are literally hundreds of decisions being made without my knowledge." As opposed to the printed schedule he received on his first visit as an outpatient, with a seamless transition from one test and appointment to the next, now he found himself as an inpatient essentially at the mercy of a large, impersonal institution. "All of a sudden, a transport person would arrive and take me for an X-ray, and I had no idea that an X-ray had been ordered. Or they would repeat blood tests in the afternoon, when I wasn't expecting to be stuck again. Then I'll tell you about a decision that just irked me. It just irked the heck out of me. The decision was made that I needed intravenous fluids, hooked up to an IV twenty-four hours a day, liter bags changed promptly at ten o'clock each morning. But then I was gaining weight, and sure enough, the bags of fluid continued to be hung there. No one questioned this. Once the decision was set into motion, there was no stopping it. I ended up gaining fifteen pounds, all fluid, and I had been in the hospital only a week." Paul asked one of the young doctors on the team if he really needed all this fluid.

"It's our protocol," he was told.

"What might seem like a very trivial decision, turned out to have a really negative effect on me." Paul's legs and thighs swelled and then his belly. "I was the victim of a rigid protocol. They want you to believe that you have control. But when you walk into a hospital environment, with these types of protocols, there is no control."

Several days later, the hematologist arrived with an informed consent document for Paul to sign. This listed the reason for the transplant and described the side effects expected with the procedure. "There is this pretense, this sort of minuet between the doctor and the patient, making believe they're involved in a rational decision, but they're not, really.

"The rules I had used in business no longer applied," Paul explained. He listed for us the underlying assumptions needed to make a medical decision in the same rational way he advised companies on a strategic decision. "The first assumption is that each aspect of the disease is well-defined and understood. Next, that all elements of information are available and considered. Third, the doctors and the patients have the same well-formulated goals. Fourth, all solutions and treatments have been considered. Fifth, every consequence of every treatment is well understood. And sixth, the outcome of every treatment can be evaluated using objective criteria."

The sixth assumption was the most problematic. "In business, the outcome can be assessed objectively, in terms of dollars. If we were to rationally assess options A, B, and C, each a particular path for the company, then to make the best decision we need to compare A, B, and C on a dollar outcome basis. That is, each outcome is measured using the same objective criterion—money." But when the doctors talked to Paul about undergoing a bone marrow transplant, he realized that these business-derived assumptions could not be applied. The nature of the outcomes could not be measured objectively.

Paul told us, "Clinical medicine is an area that moves away from clarity, an area that I think of as having higher uncertainty. You can't really make rational decisions in this world. Doctors like to have what I call a 'badge of rationality,' because it gives them authority, and they try to appear competent for the patients. It's really unsettling for the doctor to be uncertain, and even more disturbing for the patient. I keep in my head a whole list of synonyms for uncertainty: unsure, skeptical, unreliable, fickle, capricious, indecisive, controversial, vague, indefinitive. I mean, are those labels you want to apply to your doctor? So I think that even if the situation is highly uncertain, they go out of their way to appear certain, to ooze rationality."

One of the major risks of a bone marrow transplant is "graft versus host" disease. This occurs when the bone marrow from the donor, grafted into the host's body, treats the host's tissues as foreign. The new, transplanted blood cells then attack the host's skin, bowel, liver, and other organs. Paul already knew that the transplanted donor cells could attack and damage parts of his body. The consent form stated that his skin might become so inflamed that it could slough off; he could suffer intense diarrhea; his liver might fail, sending him into a coma. But the attack of the transplanted cells, "graft versus host," could be partially tempered with powerful and potentially toxic medications.

"How could I assess what it means to have graft-versus-host disease as an outcome without ever having experienced it?" Paul asked rhetorically. "So I'm thinking, How do I evaluate it? How do I measure the severity and impact on my quality of life as an individual? They told me I had a 50 percent chance of getting graft-versus-host disease, with a 10 percent chance of it affecting my liver, a 40 percent chance hurting my intestine, a 30 percent chance involving my skin. I have no way to understand what that all means."

Paul pointed out that as opposed to money, which is an objective outcome, there is no objective measure for the experience of graft-versus-host disease, either immediately or over time. "When I say over time, it means that having a complication like skin or liver or intestinal toxicity is not a static experience."

Paul went ahead with the marrow transplant. The procedure itself was successful, but he is living with graft-versus-host disease. Paul was familiar with the three methods of assigning a "utility" to your state of health—the 0 to 100 scale, the time trade-off, and the standard gamble. He echoed the views of numerous researchers that no method captures the dynamic nature of living with illness. "Some days it is better, some days it's worse. I take medications for it, so that it fluctuates in terms of severity. And, of course, I'm experiencing the side effects of those drugs. Some days they are mild, but other days not. I'm nauseated, fatigued, have no appetite. So for me to have been able to sit at point zero, looking down the pike at a bone marrow transplant and the real risk of graft-versus-host disease, and make a truly rational decision, like in economics—it just couldn't be done."

Considerable research points to the wide gulf between imagined and actual quality of life. A remarkable study assessed well-being in two groups of people: lottery winners who had just received a windfall of money and accident victims who had just become paraplegic. Not surprisingly, the two groups reported vastly different levels of well-being, with lottery winners exhilarated by their good luck and accident victims terribly depressed at their immobility.

But two years later, the levels of happiness of these markedly different groups were both similar to that of the control subjects. There are two explanations for this surprising finding. The first is the "contrast effect." We experience our current state more profoundly when we contrast it with how we were most recently. Someone who is not rich on Tuesday and wins the lottery on Wednesday profoundly experiences the sharp contrast in the immediate rise in his net worth. Similarly, a person who was dancing Saturday night and then hit by a drunk driver on the way home, waking up in the hospital on Sunday morning unable to move her legs, experiences her paralysis in a most devastating way. But over time, the lottery winners find that subsequent events, like buying a new car or taking a vacation to an exotic locale, don't have the same impact and frisson as that exhilarating moment when they won the lottery. Paraplegics experience subsequent events in an opposite way. Attending a family milestone, like a child's wedding, or competing in the wheelchair division of a marathon is experienced as a joyous triumph.

Along the same lines, many psychological studies show that we regularly underestimate our ability to adapt. People without a disability rate the "utility" or "value" of life with a particular medical problem significantly lower than those who actually live with the disability. For example, blindness is thought to be much worse by those who have sight compared with those who have lived without sight for many years. The same is true of a colostomy after bowel surgery. Most healthy people recoil at the idea of such an outcome and assign a lower "utility" or "value" than those who have one, who see their quality of life as much higher. Human beings are extraordinary in their skill at adapting, finding "value" in their lives, drawing on untapped reserves of resilience.

"I mean, the quality of my life now compared to what I had before I developed muscle disease might be considered very poor," Paul told us. "But you know, I wake up every morning and I'm happy to be here. It's great. You know, I'm just happy to be able to do what I do. When I was healthy, I probably would have said I never would want to live this way. Life is still a miracle."

Eight

End of Life

Traditionally, physicians and families shielded patients with life-threatening conditions from candid conversations about dying. Doctors or families often made decisions to continue or to stop treatment without consulting the patient. In 1983, a presidential commission released a landmark report entitled "Deciding to Forgo Life-Sustaining Treatment," which called for a change in this approach to care. The report urged doctors to speak directly with patients about CPR, intubation, and other aggressive measures that could keep a patient alive. The advance directive, or "living will," provided a framework in which patients could specify their own preferences about what care they wanted or would forgo when faced with a life-threatening disease, and such directives became widely adopted. This document also designated a family member or friend to serve as a surrogate should the patient become incapacitated and unable to make decisions for herself. Underpinning the living will was an assumption that much of the complexity and stress of making decisions about intensive treatments would be solved by specifying one's wishes in advance. But considerable research has since raised doubts about relying on advance directives.

M ary Quinn had planned every detail of her funeral down to the clothes she would wear in her casket. When she was sixty-four years old, a librarian living in Wisconsin, she had been told that she had three to six months to live. That was ten years ago. The diagnosis was cancer of the bile ducts, a tumor that rarely is cured by chemotherapy or radiation. A slim woman of medium height, with sparkling blue eyes and graying blond hair, Mary had never been seriously ill. Her parents had emigrated from Ireland and made their way to America in the aftermath of World War I. Mary and her husband were high school sweethearts, married when he was discharged from the army, and they had raised three daughters and a son. She was devoted to her family. Mary was the matriarch, running her household, and guiding the children's education. She worked in the town library, where she took particular pleasure in helping young people discover books that she believed would speak to them. A woman of deep faith, Mary attended mass every Sunday, and on Thursday evenings she prepared and served meals in the parish soup kitchen.

"She was the eternal optimist," her daughter Deidre told us. "If the house was on fire, then my mother would say, 'We'll be warm for the winter.'"

After the diagnosis of incurable biliary cancer, Mary told her family that she was ready to die: "I've had a great life." This was the way of the world, she said, a fact that everyone would someday face. But Deidre insisted on a second opinion and took Mary to another medical center, where the doctors offered an experimental therapy. After an operation that removed some of the cancer around the bile ducts, a catheter was placed, and chemotherapy was infused directly into the remaining tumor.

"It was like a miracle," Deidre told us. The cancer decreased dramatically in size. And for some eight years, the tumor didn't disappear, but it didn't grow, either. After the treatment, Mary retired from her job at the library, yet she seemed to be busier than ever. She volunteered at the local public school to assist in a reading program, organized a clothes drive each autumn at her church, and spent more time taking care of her grandchildren, lightening the load on her daughters.

But as the eighth year of remission drew to a close, she fell ill. It began gradually as discomfort in her right side, and then she developed fevers. The doctors performed blood tests and repeated her scans. The picture of her liver had changed. The doctors detected multiple new small, oval areas in her liver, which appeared to be abscesses.

Mary entered the hospital and was treated with intravenous antibiotics. The therapy seemed to improve her symptoms; her fever abated, and her energy level improved. She returned home. But after several months, the fevers and fatigue returned, and repeat tests showed more oval areas in her liver that were likely pockets of infection. Over the course of the next five months, Mary entered the hospital twice more for intravenous antibiotics. After each discharge, Deidre told us, Mary was weaker, forced to give up her volunteer activity at school, unable to stand on her feet to serve meals at church. She hardly had enough energy to read and spent most of her days in bed, dozing. Her world had begun to telescope, and Mary, still the family matriarch, gave clear guidance to Deidre and her siblings.

"She reminded us all that she did not want any heroics," Deidre recalled. "She said she was ready to die when her time came. And that she wanted to die at home, with dignity."

On her fourth admission to the hospital, intravenous antibiotics failed to bring down Mary's fever and shrink the abscesses. The doctor suggested a drainage procedure, where a needle would be placed into several of the pockets of infection and the pus drained. Mary agreed. At first the procedure seemed successful, and her fevers abated. But after several weeks at home, her temperature rose again, and she was readmitted to the hospital. A repeat scan showed that the abscesses were enlarging. Her doctors also saw what they called "shadows," and it was difficult to tell whether these dark areas in the liver were from the cancer growing or from the infection—or both. Again the medical team performed a drainage procedure, and Mary returned home.

Mary now spent nearly the entire day in bed, often dozing off after reading just a page or two of one of her favorite novels. "It seemed to us that the quality of her life was being lost," Deidre reflected. "But then, small things seemed to make her so happy to be alive." On one occasion, Deidre told us, she had baked blueberry muffins and brought them over, still warm, to Mary.

"She took a bite, and her whole face brightened. 'Oh, a muffin—look at that—with blueberries—and such blueberries!' It was as if I had painted the *Mona Lisa*, she took such pleasure in it."

This time, Mary's stay at home lasted less than a month before she was admitted once again to the hospital. Deidre arrived in the evening and sat at her bedside, reading out loud a fiction piece from a collection by one of Mary's favorite authors. Mary fell asleep during the story. Deidre sighed, then closed the book.

A few minutes later, Mary awoke. "It's getting harder and harder, Mom. How do you see things?" Deidre asked.

"I want to keep trying," Mary replied. "I want to fight."

"We were all shocked and confused by what she said." Deidre told us that she and her family were expecting that Mary would reiterate her earlier wishes and firmly decline more treatment. "But she became defiant," Deidre told us. "And she was as clear as ever. It wasn't that she was confused, or on any medication that could account for her change."

In 1995, researchers published results from a nationwide project termed the "Study to Understand Prognoses and Preferences for Outcomes and Risks of Treatment" (SUPPORT). The aim was to rigorously evaluate measures that would improve end-of-life decision making and reduce the number of patients dying in the intensive care unit, on ventilators, and in pain. There were nearly five thousand patients in the study, with a range of illnesses that often are fatal: not only widespread cancer, but also acute respiratory failure; sepsis with shutdown of multiple organs like the liver and kidneys; coma; chronic lung disease like emphysema; congestive heart failure; and cirrhosis of the liver.

Patients were randomly assigned to an intervention group or a control group. The control group of patients received the usual care. The intervention group received usual care, but in addition patients were assigned a skilled nurse. The nurse provided "timely and reliable" information to both physicians and patients about the prognosis of the illness and expected length of survival. She also helped elicit the preferences of patients and their families about whether they wanted further treatment. The researchers noted that the nurse undertook "time-consuming discussions, arranged meetings, provided information, supplied forms, and anything else to encourage the patient and family to engage in an informed and collaborative decision-making process with well-informed physicians."

The results of the study were deeply disappointing. The concerted intervention of trained nurses failed to improve end-of-life care. Specifically, the level of pain and number of days spent in the intensive care unit, in coma, or on a ventilator before death was the same in both groups. Further, researchers concluded that advance directives did not consistently improve decision making by patients and family members about end-of-life care.

What accounts for these disappointing results? Research done over the years following the SUPPORT project shows that the reason advance directives prove less useful than once thought is, in part, because a person's wishes about treatment often fluctuate over the course of an illness. Mary Quinn was far from unusual in changing her mind.

Dr. Terri Fried of Yale University, an expert in end-of-life decision making, documented how preferences change in a study of 189 patients over a two-year period. As in the SUPPORT study, these patients had conditions typically seen at the end of life: heart failure, cancer, and chronic lung diseases like emphysema. Although many had been hospitalized in the previous year and some had even been in the intensive care unit, most of the patients rated their current quality of life as good. These patients were repeatedly interviewed about their wishes to undergo medical interventions like intubation and being placed on a ventilator and their willingness to undergo a treatment that would prevent death but might, or might not, leave them bedridden or with significant cognitive disability.

Nearly half of the patients were inconsistent in their wishes about their treatments. Although more people whose health got worse over the two-year period showed shifting preferences, even those whose health was stable changed their wishes. Completing a living will or advance directive had no effect on whether they maintained or shifted their initial thoughts about what therapies they wanted.

For that reason, Dr. Rebecca L. Sudore of the University of California at San Francisco, with Dr. Fried of Yale, wrote in the *Annals of Internal Medicine* in 2010 that the "planning" in so-called advance care planning needs to be redefined: "The traditional objective of advance care planning has been to have patients make treatment decisions in advance of serious illness so that clinicians can attempt to provide care consistent with their goals." But such advance directives "frequently do not . . . improve clinician and surrogate knowledge of patient preferences." The "traditional objective of making advance decisions," setting out a path that physicians and family members can follow in order to honor the earlier wishes of the patient, is a "fundamentally flawed" objective. Dr. Muriel Gillick, a geriatrician at Harvard Medical School and researcher in end-of-life care, wrote that same year in the *New England Journal of Medicine*, "Despite the prodigious effort devoted to designing, legislating, and studying advance directives, the consensus of medical ethicists, researchers in health care services, and palliative care physicians is that the directives have been a resounding failure."

Patients deviate from their own advance directives because, like Mary, they often can't imagine what they will want and how much they can endure when their condition shifts from healthy to sick and then to even sicker. As Sudore and Fried noted, "Individuals have difficulty predicting what they would want in future circumstances because these predictions do not reflect the current medical, emotional, or social context."

Why is it so difficult for us when we are healthy to imagine the future under difficult circumstances? Sudore and Fried suggest that "one major determinant of changing preferences is adaptability. Patients often cannot envision being able to cope with disability and report the desire to forgo aggressive treatments in such states. However, once patients experience those health states, they are often more willing to accept even invasive treatments with limited benefits."

In addition to underestimating our ability to adapt, two other cognitive influences are at work. First is focalism. This refers to a narrow focus on what will change in one's life while ignoring how much will stay the same and can still be enjoyed. Mary originally thought that life wouldn't be worth living if she was bedridden. And indeed when she became ill, her family, being healthy, viewed the quality of her life as so poor that it didn't seem worth continuing. But Mary found that she could still take tremendous pleasure in even the smallest aspects of living, the taste of her favorite muffin, served warm, prepared by her devoted daughter. She wanted to go on living, despite once imagining that she would not.

Second is what we term "buffering." People generally fail to recognize the degree to which their coping mechanisms will buffer them from emotional suffering. This is because such coping mechanisms are largely unconscious processes. Denial, rationalization, humor, intellectualization, and compartmentalization are all coping mechanisms that can help make life endurable, even at times fulfilling, when we are ill.

The will to live, under even worsening conditions, is very powerful.

Mary's fevers continued. A repeat scan of her liver showed that the abscesses had grown larger, their walls thicker, and more "shadows" filled their centers. The resident doctor showed Deidre and her family the images. Deidre asked the resident if this could be a growing tumor rather than just infection. "We really don't know," he replied.

In the early evening on the second day of Mary's treatment, a hospitalist came to her room. Hospitalists are physicians who are trained in inpatient medicine, and over the past few years they have increasingly assumed the care of people who are admitted to the hospital. Deidre and her father were at the bedside when she entered, a young woman in her early thirties. "How are you feeling today, Mrs. Quinn?" she asked.

Mary responded, "Not so well today, Doctor."

"I'm sorry to hear that. You know, we are trying to treat your infection, but we don't seem to be making progress," the doctor said. "We need to know how much more you want done."

Deidre's father looked away, and Deidre saw his eyes well with tears.

"Why can't you treat my infection?" Mary asked.

The doctor explained that Mary had received multiple different antibiotics over the past several months, and the antibiotics weren't working anymore. She continued that they weren't sure whether the new ones they were now administering would succeed since the bacteria may have changed and become resistant to the drugs. Furthermore, the antibiotics might not be getting into the abscesses.

Mary listened quietly, then said, "Can you drain the abscess again? That helped before."

"Yes, we could try that, but it may not work," she responded. "From the scans, it also seems as if the cancer may be starting to grow again," she added.

Mary's face took on a tight and determined look; she fixed her gaze on the physician. "I want to be treated."

"Okay, then," she said. "We will keep going."

"It seemed like Mom was going against everything that she had told us before." The family was distraught and confused by this change, Deidre told us. "She had said no heroic measures, and that she wanted to die with dignity, not be in the hospital, to spend her last days at home. Now, she was agreeing to more procedures, more needles."

The morning after Mary told the hospitalist that she wanted to keep going, her oncologist visited her. This specialist had treated her over the years and knew the family well. He and Mary were very fond of each other.

"How is that novel?" the oncologist asked, picking up a book from her nightstand. "It got great reviews."

"I'm too exhausted to read," Mary replied. "But I'm hoping to catch up once I go home."

Deidre was sitting near the head of the bed. Mary turned toward her daughter. "Don't forget that Sean's birthday is next week," Mary said. "Dee, pick up that book we talked about. He's expecting it from Grandma." Deidre said she would.

"Mary, I heard that you're thinking about your wishes, what makes sense for you now," the oncologist said. Like many oncologists, he was trained in what the end-of-life specialists term "the conversation." He had acquired skills to gently but clearly focus his patients on understanding their circumstances and better delineating their preferences.

"Mary, I understand that you said you want to continue with antibiotics for now."

Mary nodded. "Yes. I do."

"I understand your wishes. But if circumstances changed, like you were to go into a coma, would you want us to sustain you?"

Mary didn't answer right away. Her eyes turned toward Deidre and then focused back on the oncologist.

"No. I wouldn't want that."

"Would you want us to keep you on a ventilator if you couldn't breathe on your own?"

Mary shook her head. "No."

"At that point you'd want us to focus on comfort, to make sure that there was no pain, and that everything was, as you told me before, dignified."

Mary's eyes filled with tears. Deidre stood up, took a tissue from the bedside table, and wiped her mother's eyes.

"I want to live," Mary said. "I want you to keep trying to get rid of these infections."

"I understand. We will do our best," the oncologist assured her.

Deidre walked with him into the corridor, out of Mary's earshot. "I can't believe that she wants to keep going," Deidre said. Mary's medical team had proposed again attempting to drain the largest abscesses and also to obtain a biopsy to assess how much cancer might be present in the lesions. "Do you think she should do this?" Deidre asked.

"I think it's worth her undergoing the procedure, so that we can find out where we stand," the oncologist said. "If there is extensive regrowth of cancer, this will help tell us whether we should push on or not. I'll come back tomorrow and we'll all talk again."

Not long after the oncologist left, the gastroenterology fellow came to obtain an informed consent for the procedure. He paused, looking at Mary's wasted form, dwarfed by the hospital bed. Deidre said, "You know, she was a librarian for forty years. Just an amazing woman." The doctor nodded. "She raised four children, three daughters and a son," Deidre continued, "and now she has seven grandchildren. One of them has a birthday next week."

Deidre told us, "I always wanted to bring a human face to people about who she was. This is my mother, a person and not just a patient. Because it can get just to be that way, patients all hooked up to machines, nurses and doctors doing a job."

Not long after the young doctor left with the form signed by Mary, a case manager entered the room. Mary was sleeping, so the case manager and Deidre moved into the hall. "I'm arranging the transfer for Mrs. Quinn to a rehabilitation facility," the woman said.

Deidre was shocked. No one had ever mentioned discharging Mary from the hospital and transferring her to another facility. "My mother doesn't want to go to rehab," Deidre told her. "We want to bring Mom home." Deidre told us that the manager said flatly, "'Well, you'll never be able to care for her at home.' And I said, 'Well, we're going to figure something out.'

"Mom had told my father that she wanted to die at home," Deidre recalled. "This news would have made my mother even more upset than she already was. We decided we didn't have to talk about it right then."

A half hour after the news about transferring Mary to a rehabilitation facility, a transport person arrived, saying, "Hi, Mrs. Quinn, I'm here to take you downstairs for your procedure."

"That day, I felt everything slipping away from any sort of rational progression," Deidre said. "All sorts of things were happening that we weren't aware of. And it felt like we couldn't get a handle on who was in charge or what was going on. It seemed like decisions were being made automatically."

Deidre had another observation to share with us: "There just is this massive bureaucracy that hospitals have become. It seems so crazy, you are sort of caught in a whirlwind. And sometimes it's like, 'What's going on here?' And there were times when there was just no clear communication, when everything felt so out of control."

Mary was taken to the procedure suite. She'd been given a mild sedative, and she soon fell asleep. The liver specialist cleaned her skin and then, under ultrasound guidance, he inserted a needle into one of the large cavities. Almost immediately, Mary began to gasp for air. The doctor put an oxygen mask on her face, then listened to her heart and lungs. Within short order, the reason for her respiratory distress became clear: He had punctured her right lung when he inserted the needle into her liver. Although uncommon, this is a known risk of this procedure.

The liver specialist checked her orders; there was no "Do Not

Intubate" directive. The code team was paged—residents came rushing in. A breathing tube was placed into Mary's trachea. A surgical resident sliced between her ribs and inserted a chest tube to reexpand her lungs. Mary was rushed to the intensive care unit.

Deidre, her father, and siblings were awake all night in the family room next to the ICU. The nurses told them that Mary had not woken up since the lung collapse. It was still unclear why she hadn't regained consciousness. Shortly after noon, the oncologist visited and told the Quinn family that the liver biopsy showed "extensive cancer."

"I'm so sorry this complication happened," the oncologist said. "But I think the procedure was important, that it was worth doing, because now we know where we stand."

Deidre told us that her father felt "paralyzed," and although he was the health proxy, he was so distraught that he could hardly speak.

Mr. Quinn couldn't stay and watch his wife die. "It was too hard for Dad," Deidre said, "so I told my brother to take him home. Not to worry. We girls would be with her." One of Deidre's sisters went to her car and got the rosary beads that Mary had given her as a child. Another sister had brought the handkerchief that Mary had embroidered for her and she had carried all through her growing years.

"It's funny how you revert," Deidre said. "We all sat there with Mom. It was as if we were all back in elementary school together. My sister started saying the rosary, and my other sister held on tight to the hanky. We all grew up in the same house, the three of us shared a room, and we were all there together.

"We decided together to take her off the ventilator," Deidre told us. "Now that we knew that the cancer was back in force and she was unconscious. The conversation with the oncologist helped clarify things for us."

Mary was still unconscious when she was taken off the ventilator. Within a minute, her chest began to heave and she was gasping for air.

The nurse gave Mary morphine. "If you had asked me five years ago, could I be in the room and watch my mother die, I would have said, No. But somehow I found I was able to do that, even though it was horrific. When they took the tube out, I heard those noises, Mom gasping, her arms flailing. It was so horrible. I could do nothing but weep. But that was very cathartic. So that surprised me on a personal level." Over the course of several hours, the gasping slowed. Mary died just as the sun was setting.

After Mary's death, Deidre spent much time reflecting on what had happened. We asked her if another loved one became seriously ill, would she handle things any differently from the way things had gone with her mother? "I want to shout out and say, 'Yes!'" Deidre replied. "We thought we had had the conversation, but we hadn't. We thought we agreed on no heroics—that everything would be clear. But it wasn't. It was such a struggle for me, and looking back, I feel guilty that I never had an open conversation with Mom about palliative care, instead of one more procedure to try and poke a hole in her liver, and drain it and get rid of the infection. My biggest struggle personally is that that kind of conversation was never held."

A study published in 2010 in the *New England Journal of Medicine* evaluated the potential benefit of early introduction of what is called "palliative care." This involved "specific attention" to assessing "physical and psychosocial symptoms, establishing goals of care, assisting with decision making regarding treatment, and coordinating care on the basis of the individual needs of the patient." All these patients had newly diagnosed metastatic lung cancer. They were treated at Massachusetts General Hospital but weren't hospitalized. Rather, they were living at home. The patients were randomly assigned either to receive usual care or to receive usual care and palliative care. Those assigned to the palliative care group met at least monthly with specialized physicians or nurses. The results of the research showed that patients receiving palliative care chose less aggressive therapies but nonetheless lived longer, some two to three months, and had somewhat better quality of life. In the editorial accompanying the article, Drs. Amy Kelley and Diane Meier of Mount Sinai Medical Center in New York noted the "salutary effect" of additional time with and attention from physicians, nurses, and other health care professionals.

The need to provide more individual attention and spend more time with very sick patients will collide with a modern medical system that increasingly rewards "efficiency." Prominent health policy planners, and even some physicians, envision the hospital and its clinic as a factory and assert that medical care should be delivered in an industrialized fashion. Visits with patients are shaved down to a few minutes; conversations are structured to meet standardized protocols and quality measures. But the difficult and often changing decisions patients make about what and how much more to do in the midst of a life-threatening condition are not "products" that "efficiently" roll off an assembly line. Guiding a patient and her family as she nears the end of her life is neither an easy nor an efficient process. It takes time and effort because it is not direct, not linear; it involves much back-and-forth discussion, often without coming to a decision or, after deciding, reversing that choice and then later changing choices again. This new medical system might be more efficient in delivering certain types of care, but it often ends up not caring for the patient.

Time isn't the only barrier to helping a very sick patient understand her condition and clarify her wishes about treatments. Deidre considered how many issues made it difficult to have a conversation with Mary about palliative care. "I think we never had a real talk about dying because she wanted to protect my father. She was the matriarch, she was the strong one, and somehow I think she was afraid that if it was out in the open, he just couldn't handle it. But I also think it was her will to live. And her faith. She just wasn't ready to die."

Mary Quinn changed her wishes about intensive measures during the course of her illness, like half the patients in the Yale study by Dr. Terri Fried. But the other half held fast. Like those patients, Ruth Adler did not change her mind.

R uth Adler had also planned her funeral down to the last detail. She had selected the rabbi who would preside, the psalms that would be read, the music that would be sung. That was also ten years ago. Now seventy-five years old, a petite woman with a crown of thick white hair in a youthful pageboy cut, she lived just outside Washington, D.C. A homemaker who was active in her synagogue and community, Ruth was long familiar with medical illness. As a child, she'd had kidney ailments that required repeated surgery. Her youth was marked by many months in the hospital and winters with cousins in Florida in the belief that the warm climate would help her heal. As an adult, Ruth ate a healthy and balanced diet, was meticulous in how she took medications, and believed in doing the maximum to avoid problems. Her daughter, Naomi, told us, "My mom was all about maintenance and prevention. She always wanted to do everything right."

At the age of thirty, Ruth was diagnosed with breast cancer. She underwent what was then the most aggressive therapy, a radical mastectomy, followed by intense radiation treatments that burned her chest wall. In addition, both ovaries and uterus were removed. Her breast cancer never returned, but she was left with burned, scarred skin on her chest wall.

Ten years ago, at the age of sixty-five, Ruth fainted while shopping in a local supermarket. She was taken to the emergency room and found to have aortic stenosis, a narrowing of the aortic valve in the heart, which limits the amount of blood that can be pumped out to the brain and other organs. Ruth was evaluated by a cardiologist and a cardiac surgeon. Both agreed that her condition required open heart surgery to replace the diseased aortic valve with an artificial valve. But the operation was even more risky than usual because the incision would have to be made through the irradiated skin and might not heal.

Naomi told us, "She knew it was serious surgery, and she prepared the family by saying that she didn't want to live debilitated in any way." Before the operation, Ruth designated her husband, Naomi's stepfather, as her health proxy. She also drew up an advance directive, specifying that there were to be no heroic measures and no effort at resuscitation.

After Ruth's surgery, her doctors strongly advised her to go to a rehabilitation facility for a few months, but she adamantly refused. "She said she won't ever go to rehab. That was totally against how she wanted to live," Naomi said. Ruth insisted on going directly home to recuperate. The incision over her breastbone never fully healed. Ruth consulted with her cardiac surgeon and a plastic surgeon, who agreed that she needed to have reconstruction, with a muscle flap taken from her back and grafted onto the skin that hadn't healed.

"Mom flat-out refused," Naomi said. Instead, she followed a naturalism orientation. "She did positive imaging, focusing her mind on the area that wouldn't heal," Naomi recounted. "And a friend of hers went to a special beach and brought back seawater that Mom bathed the area in. After a few months, it closed."

Never one to mince words, Ruth told Naomi that she was "tired from all the surgery and hospitalizations and never wanted to go to the hospital again." She wanted to do everything possible to stay healthy enough to be present for joyous occasions with her family. But she was clear in her limits.

When Ruth was seventy-four, she went on a long-planned trip to China. She was fascinated by the East, was thrilled to tour the Forbidden City in Beijing and climb to the top of the Great Wall. When she returned home, she told Naomi that she was happy she'd made the journey, but she just wasn't feeling well. She had developed a persistent nagging pain in her chest. Her primary care doctor ordered X-rays. A wire placed to close the breastbone at the time of her heart surgery had now loosened.

"After that, she had good days and bad days," Naomi said. "She struggled to live with the pain. She did not like pain medication, not at all; she said it made her feel druggy."

Over the next year, Naomi found Ruth spending much of her time in bed. "This was not my mother," Naomi told us. Ruth was the one who organized events for the sisterhood at the synagogue. She also kept track of members of the congregation who were ill, writing them notes wishing them a rapid recovery; if she knew the person, she would call and offer words of encouragement. But Ruth was finding it harder and harder to keep up these activities. Then, in early winter, Naomi called on a Saturday afternoon to check on her mother.

"I feel terrible," Ruth said. "I couldn't go to shul. I need to see my doctor."

Naomi reminded her that it was the weekend. If she needed to see a doctor, she'd have to go to the emergency room.

"Then take me," Ruth replied.

Naomi was shocked, "because I knew how much my mother hated the hospital. Whatever was going on had to be serious."

Naomi picked up Ruth at her home ten minutes away. Ruth gave her a weak hug and planted a kiss on her cheek, as she always did when they met. Naomi tried to keep one eye on Ruth and the other on the road as she drove to the hospital.

"I don't know what's wrong, but something is really wrong with my mother," Naomi told the triage nurse. In short order, Ruth was taken into an examination room, where her blouse and slacks were removed and replaced by a hospital gown. The nurse checked her blood pressure, then took it again.

Ruth was sitting on an examination table, staring intently at the nurse. "Why are you checking my pressure again?" Ruth asked.

"You might feel better lying down," the nurse said. "Your blood pressure is extremely low." The upper number is normally 120; Ruth's pressure barely reached 70.

Naomi retreated into a corner as the room quickly filled with medical personnel. A technician placed an IV line into Ruth's arm, while EKG leads were applied to her chest, arms, and legs. She was then examined by a young doctor who introduced himself as the ER attending physician. "I feel terrible," Ruth told him.

The doctor asked, "Are you having any pain?"

"Not really. Well, I do have this pain over my breastbone, but I have had that for months," Ruth said. "I just feel awful, so awful."

The doctor explained to Ruth that she was on the cusp of going into shock. "You don't look sick, but you are," he said. "And we need to know your wishes if something would happen, if your blood pressure were to fall even lower."

"I have an advance care directive. My daughter can give you that, although I think it's already in my medical record," Ruth said. "And my husband is my health care proxy." She paused and then trained her eyes directly on the doctor's. "I do not want any artificial assistance, none at all."

Ruth turned to Naomi and said, "Are you ready to lose me?"

Naomi's eyes filled with tears, and she gripped her mother's hand.

"Are you ready for me to be gone?" Ruth asked.

Naomi was mute. She began to tremble.

"Are you okay with this, with my wishes?"

Naomi later told us, "It was so confusing to me to have her talking like this." She explained that her mother was awake, alert, answering the doctor's questions in full and coherent sentences. "And there was no diagnosis."

Ruth was transferred directly from the ER to the ICU. It turned out that she had an infection in her blood—sepsis. The doctors infused saline and high doses of antibiotics. Despite this treatment, her blood pressure hovered around 90. Over the next few hours, her breathing became more labored. The doctors in the ICU explained that sepsis can interfere with lung function. Furthermore, Ruth had severe osteoporosis, likely from having had her ovaries removed at a very young age. Despite taking calcium and vitamin D supplements and other medications regularly, her vertebrae had gradually weakened and collapsed. Now, bent over from the changes in her spine, it was hard for her to fully expand her lungs.

Over the next twenty-four hours, Ruth became weaker and weaker. At one point, as the nurse was bathing her mother, Naomi saw a small spot of pus over Ruth's breastbone.

"My mother was an immaculately kept woman," Naomi told us. "I looked at the bra that she had worn and saw that it was stained from pus. I pointed this out to the nurse. I didn't know if she had seen it." It turned out that this was the source of her infection, because bacteria had migrated from her skin to her sternum and then to her blood.

A senior ICU physician came to talk with Naomi and her stepfather. He explained that Ruth was likely to tire from the effort of breathing and wouldn't be able to keep breathing effectively without the aid of a ventilator.

"I know you have an advance directive," he said to Ruth, "but we would like to put you on a ventilator as a temporary measure, until we clear the infection."

Ruth shook her head no. "I don't want to be a vegetable," she declared. "I want to be alive and active, or gone."

The doctor reiterated that the intervention would last only until the infection could be controlled. As soon as the antibiotics took effect and her blood pressure and oxygen rose to safe ranges, they would take her off the ventilator. Ruth refused again.

Naomi and her stepfather accompanied the physician into the hall outside the room.

"She'll probably die if she doesn't agree to this," he said.

"I understand," Naomi replied. "I'll do everything I can to try and convince her."

Naomi returned to the room and spoke again with her mother. But Ruth remained adamant. "I don't want to be on a breathing machine," she said. "And I know where this can lead. If they need to keep me on it, then they'll transfer me to some chronic care facility. I don't want to live in rehab. You know that I want to be alive and active or gone."

An hour later, a middle-aged nurse who had been attending to Ruth came in.

"I'm just going to straighten up a little here," the nurse said. She took away a cup of water and prepared a new one with a fresh straw. Naomi's husband had brought pictures of the grandchildren, which were arranged on the table next to her bed. "Beautiful children," the nurse said, looking at the photographs. Ruth nodded and smiled.

"You know, my father was in a similar situation to yours," the nurse said to Ruth and Naomi. "He was very sick, and had made it clear to us that he didn't want to live if it meant being sustained artificially." The nurse paused. "He had a problem with his heart. The doctors said his heart would improve, but they needed to make sure he was getting enough oxygen to let it heal." The nurse told them that her father ultimately agreed to be placed on the ventilator, and after a few days, he was able to come off. "I saw him last weekend and he looked great. He wouldn't be with us now if he hadn't made that choice." This story had a profound impact on Naomi, as stories of hope often do for people in dire circumstances. Such narratives are an example of the powerful effect of availability.

After the nurse left, Naomi sat next to her mother. "Please, Mom," she said. "Please consider this. I'll respect whatever you choose, but it's only for a short while. Please."

Ruth didn't answer. As the afternoon wore on, her breathing became even more labored. In the early evening, her primary care doctor arrived. He had cared for her for more than a decade, and they had grown close. Her visits to him were never brief; she often lingered, talking to him not only about her medical problems, but about her grandchildren and her activities at her synagogue.

"Ruth, we've talked many times about your wishes," her doctor said. "And I am fully on board. I know the limits you set. But what we are recommending now is only temporary. Not more than a few days at most, in all likelihood."

A heavy silence filled the room.

"Think about it again," he said as he left.

The nurse who had told Ruth about her father came by to say that her shift was ending. "I hope you change your mind," she said.

Ruth's husband had been with her at the hospital since the early morning. Naomi sent him home for dinner and a shower. She sat at the bedside, refusing to leave even to get a sandwich for supper. Around ten p.m., Ruth began to gasp for breath. Naomi pressed a button for assistance.

A young doctor quickly came in, examined Ruth, and said that her blood pressure was falling.

"You need to be intubated now," the doctor said. "We need to get you on the ventilator."

Ruth was sitting bolt upright in bed. "I need . . . five minutes . . . to think about it."

"You may not have five minutes," the doctor replied.

"I am not . . . going to be . . . pressured by you," Ruth gasped. "I need to call my husband."

Naomi dialed the number.

"I love you," Ruth told her husband. "Good-bye."

Naomi started to cry.

Drs. Sudore and Fried, in their article in the *Annals of Internal Medicine* in 2010, posed the following scenario: Consider a patient with lung cancer who cannot be cured but who might live for two years or more. She has prepared an advance directive specifying "no heroic measures" and "no artificial interventions to sustain life." She then develops transient heart failure. Here, her immediate prognosis is based on her cardiac function, not on the longer-term issue of her cancer. The heart condition is treatable, but if it goes untreated, fluid will build up in the lungs, preventing enough oxygen from reaching the vital organs. To survive, the patient must be intubated and placed on a ventilator for perhaps one week. Does this qualify as a "heroic measure"? Does briefly going on a ventilator to treat a transient heart condition contradict the stated wish of "no artificial intervention"? To be sure, the expected course may be quite different from what ultimately occurs. Patients cannot anticipate every twist and turn in their condition. Perhaps the patient with lung cancer and transient heart failure will develop pneumonia and have to be kept on the ventilator for a longer period of time, or the heart failure will prove to be not temporary but a more permanent problem. Do you then discontinue the artificial life support? And if so, when? There are no definitive answers because the prognosis in such situations is unclear.

Doctors and nurses are trained to save lives—and saving a life is one of the most fulfilling acts for caregivers. Without clear instructions from the patient or surrogates not to do so, the "default option" is to do everything we can to save a patient's life. In the SUPPORT project, specialized research nurses tried to give patients and their surrogates accurate information about a prognosis to help guide their choices about accepting or declining intensive treatments. But it is difficult to do so in cases like Ruth's, where the condition is changing rapidly and each of the underlying problems—infection, weakened lungs, failing heart—may or may not be remedied with further treatment.

The limits written in Ruth's advance directive were explicit and incorporated views about what treatment was worthwhile in light of her previous experiences with kidney disease and heart surgery. However, at this point in her illness, the doctors believed that Ruth's condition was treatable and that she could regain a healthy and active life if she agreed to this temporary intervention. They felt that holding strictly to the wishes in her advance directive was not in her best interests. Yet without her explicit permission, they couldn't treat her.

"Okay," Ruth said. "I'll do it."

Ruth's blood pressure rose as her oxygen levels improved on the ventilator. But her fevers continued. The doctor in the ICU found Naomi and showed her Ruth's CT scan. "Can you see the wire there?" he asked as he walked her through the images on the computer screen. She saw a loop of metal that seemed to be suspended within the bone.

"I couldn't believe how mangled and loose the wire was. It was undone," Naomi told us. "When I saw the images, I understood a lot more about my mother's physical health."

The doctor explained that "there is a deep infection in the bone, called osteomyelitis. The bacteria track along the wire, which makes it difficult for the antibiotics to clear the infection."

This infection would not be readily eradicated with intravenous antibiotics. The doctor told Naomi that surgery was required to remove the wire and take out the fragments of bone seeded with bacteria. This would leave a gaping hole in Ruth's breastbone. Then a second operation would be required to repair the bone and close the skin.

Later that day, the infectious disease specialist arrived. She took Naomi and her stepfather to a quiet room next to the ICU. Naomi told us, "She was very honest. She said Mom was not doing well, and she couldn't beat this, even with surgery."

Not long after the infectious disease specialist left, a thoracic surgeon arrived to evaluate Ruth. After he reviewed the CT scan and examined her, he also met with Naomi and her stepfather. "He was completely confident," Naomi recalled. "He told us in no uncertain terms, 'We can do this.' Even though he explained that moving her to the operating room was a risk in itself, the surgeon said he was sure that he could successfully remove the wire and take out the infected bone." Naomi paused and then said, "We were getting mixed messages. It was confusing."

Ruth's surrogates, her husband and Naomi, were caught in a clash of conflicting expert opinions about treatment and prognosis: The infectious disease specialist predicted that Ruth would ultimately die from her infection, while the thoracic surgeon asserted that she could be cured with an operation. As illness becomes more severe and choices must be made with greater urgency, decisional conflict becomes acute. Painful dilemmas for patients and surrogates are frequent, whether it be differing opinions about the success or failure of a particular treatment or the patient's overall prognosis. This provides further insight into why the SUPPORT research might not have succeeded by offering "enhanced communication." Communication per se doesn't necessarily resolve differing opinions or reduce stark uncertainties in predicting the outcome of an operation like the one Ruth faced.

Naomi asked the surgeon about the skin, burned from radiation and now weeping pus. "We'll put a sponge in, and later do a flap procedure to reconstruct the area." The surgeon emphasized that it was imperative to perform the procedure as soon as possible. "I've scheduled her tentatively for tomorrow," he said.

Naomi told us, "We had to decide quickly. This could possibly save her."

She and her stepfather spent nearly two hours discussing the decision. "We ultimately said no," Naomi explained, "because if my mom woke up with the knowledge that we had committed her to a surgery that she had previously refused, she would have been very angry."

Late in the evening, Ruth dozed off, and the resident in the intensive care unit told Naomi that it was fine to go home. But in the middle of the night she received a call from the resident. Ruth had developed atrial fibrillation. As we discussed previously, this is an abnormal heart rhythm that can both reduce the output of blood to the tissues and cause clots to form, which could lead to a stroke. The ICU doctor wanted to know if Ruth should be cardioverted, a procedure where an electric shock is applied over the chest wall and transmitted to the heart to return the disturbed rhythm to normal.

Ruth's health proxy was Naomi's stepfather, and she reminded the doctor of this. When the doctor called him, he said, "Thank you for letting me know. But we are a party of two. Naomi and I decide together. We will call you back in a few minutes." They spoke briefly, and he asked her to call the doctor back and give their permission to go ahead with the cardioversion.

"Okay," the doctor said when Naomi called him. "But we're not getting clear direction from your family about what kinds of measures to take. You're not being consistent."

Naomi knew he was right. But it was hard to know what was consistent with her mother's wishes. She and her stepfather believed an electric shock was a temporary intervention, one that didn't seem to be "heroic" or "artificially sustaining" her. On the other hand, her mother might not see it that way.

The telephone rang again. The doctor told Naomi that the atrial fibrillation had resolved on its own, and there was no need to cardiovert Ruth. "But it may happen again," the doctor warned, "and we don't always have the time to call you."

Naomi recalled that "this was helpful. It really put into focus for us how we had to be explicit, and try to set up a process and rules that anticipated these kinds of questions.

"I knew that in the future I had to say no," Naomi told us. But she was still shaken by the burden of this decision, even while sharing it with her stepfather.

Naomi and her stepfather agreed about Ruth's care. But there are frequently several family members gathered around the bedside of a severely ill patient, and they may disagree about what treatments are best for their loved one. They are each trying to reconcile their wish to do everything possible for the patient and the terrible fear that they may simply be prolonging his or her suffering before an inevitable end. It isn't surprising that family members or other surrogates are often not of one mind. This diversity of opinion may also account for the results from the SUPPORT research: Giving family members information does not automatically generate consensus.

The next day, Naomi and her stepfather called Ruth's primary care doctor. "He agreed that 'No' would be my mother's wish," Naomi told us. "Ultimately, we had to honor my mother's wishes, even though they were not what we wanted."

While the primary care doctor didn't try to negotiate with Ruth, her husband did. Each morning, he sat by her bedside and spoke to her, trying to inspire her to continue to fight. Nearly a week had passed since the tube had been placed in her trachea. Ruth was awake and alert, and although her hand trembled, she could write a few words on a notepad. At other times, Naomi was able to read her lips as she tried to mouth words around the tube. Naomi felt acutely aware of her mother's mental clarity. "Her brain was completely alert, but her body was compromised," Naomi told us. "Everything my mother feared was happening to her."

The doctors explained that her tube couldn't stay in the trachea much longer than a week, since it might irreparably damage the airway tissue. "Today is the day," the doctor said. "We will take the tube out and hope she can breathe on her own."

As soon as the tube was removed, Ruth began gasping for breath. "She was arched forward, her arms reaching out like someone trying to draw in air from a window."

The doctor put on an oxygen mask, hoping that this would suffice. "It's not working," he said. "We have to put the tube back."

Ruth couldn't speak but shook her head repeatedly—no, no, no—and curled her lips. But then she moved her head back, closed her eyes, and did not fight when the tube was reinserted into her trachea. She fell asleep, but when she awoke back on the ventilator, she was angry.

Over the next two days, the doctors tried to have Ruth sit up in a chair, hoping that her lungs might more efficiently capture the oxygen if her chest was at a higher angle. "My mom hated being moved," Naomi told us. "Just getting from the bed to the chair was torture."

The doctors explained that the tube in her throat had been in place too long and must be removed. If she still couldn't breathe on her own, the next step would be a tracheostomy, a procedure where a hole is made in the neck and a tube inserted directly into the trachea rather than through the mouth. Then she could be discharged to a rehabilitation facility. Once she recovered, the tracheostomy could be closed, and she would breathe on her own.

Ruth wrote in her trembling script, "NO." She refused the tracheostomy. She would never go to a rehab facility.

The ICU doctor told Naomi, "We need to see again if she can breathe on her own. If she can't, she will need the tracheostomy." So later that day, the ICU team removed the tube and placed her on an oxygen mask. Her primary care physician stood by the bedside.

Within seconds, Ruth lunged forward, gasping for air. "We need to do that tracheostomy," the ICU doctor said.

Ruth shook her head no. "If you make that choice, you won't live," he said bluntly.

"No," Ruth said in a reedy whisper.

Naomi saw the shock register on the faces of the doctor and nurse. Ruth's husband threw himself on her bed. "Please, Ruth, please," he cried, sobbing.

Ruth shook her head.

The doctor fitted the oxygen mask over Ruth's face. She continued to labor in her breathing through the day. Her primary care doctor promised to check in on her periodically. Naomi and her stepfather sat by Ruth's bed. Naomi said, "Mom, is there anything I can do for you?" Leaning in close to her mother, she tried to read her mother's lips. "Iced tea?" Naomi asked. She knew her mother loved this drink.

The same nurse who had convinced Ruth to go on the ventilator when she told the story of her father brought a glass to the bedside. Naomi lifted the glass of iced tea to Ruth's mouth. She took a small sip, laid her head back against the pillow, and closed her eyes.

"I stayed awake all night with her so she would not be alone. In the morning, the doctor told me it would be okay to go home, freshen up, and come back in an hour or two. They would call if anything changed."

As Naomi stepped out of the shower, the phone was ringing. It was the hospital. "Your mother's failing. You need to come in," a nurse said.

"At the end, it was two minutes," Naomi said. "They told me she had passed just two minutes before I entered the room." She paused. "I think it is easier for people to leave when their loved ones are not in the room. For my mother to leave us was very hard. She was so brave. After Mom was gone, I got in bed with her and I cried."

We spoke with Naomi again a year after Ruth's death. She reflected on the experience. "My mother was always very clear about what she wanted. As hard as it was at the end, I felt that we honored her wishes. But sometimes it wasn't clear if what the doctors were proposing would fit with my mother's wishes or not. I had to keep thinking, Is this treatment consistent with my mother's wishes if it is only temporary? Should she consider this option? It wasn't always obvious. It was sometimes very confusing for me."

While Ruth Adler was consistent in what she wanted, that consistency didn't make it any easier for her surrogates to know if a particular intervention respected her advance directive. This dilemma isn't unusual, as Dr. Terri Fried and John O'Leary of Yale found when they interviewed sixty-four bereaved family members in Connecticut. The challenge was particularly great when the patients suffered from heart or lung disease. While families usually accept that diseases like metastatic cancer are ultimately terminal, they find it harder to imagine that modern technologies like ventilators and bypass machines cannot save loved ones who have heart or lung disease. As a culture, our technology bias is powerful here: The heart is, in essence, a pump; the lungs are bellows. There must be an engineering solution to problems of these organs.

Fried and O'Leary's study recounted an experience that echoed that of the Adler family. In this case, the physician also told the patient's daughter that her mother must be intubated or she would die. By going on the ventilator, the doctor said, her mother would get her strength back and her lungs would clear. "My mother wouldn't have it," the daughter reported. "She said, 'I'm not going through that.' I said, 'Do you understand that you are going to die?' And she said, 'I'm ready to die.'" Like Ruth, the woman in Connecticut held to the set limits in her advance directive, even though they clashed with what the doctor thought best and what her family wanted.

Beyond advance directives, what can be done to improve decision making during critical illness?

Certain states like Oregon, New York, and North Carolina have tried to refine the advance directive by having the patient specify what treatments he or she wants at the time of hospital admission: full CPR, or short of CPR, antibiotics, intravenous fluids, comfort measures like oxygen and pain medications. Physicians then write orders in the patient's chart about each intervention. While this may be helpful, experts in palliative care emphasize that there are no shortcuts around serious, time-consuming, and emotionally charged conversations between the patient, loved ones, and doctors, like those the Quinn and Adler families had. Such conversations do not follow one script and sometimes take sharp detours. But repeated communication can bring clarity to the complex choices that all of us may one day face. An advance directive, or living will, is the beginning, not the end, of expressing our wishes.

Nine

When the Patient
Can't Decide

The principle of autonomy dictates that the patient has the right to choose or to refuse any offered treatments. But when you are ill and in the hospital, you may be least able to make these choices. Studies indicate that as many as 40 percent of adult hospitalized patients are receiving sedating drugs, confused, or even comatose and therefore incapable of making their own decisions about therapy. Since incapacitated patients can't actively communicate their wishes, family members or other surrogates must make decisions for them. Some surrogates may want to assert autonomy on the patient's behalf; other surrogates may want to relinquish control to the physician. During the course of a complex illness, changing circumstances may shift the role of decision maker back and forth between surrogate and doctor.

O mar Akil had never really thought about being sick. A forty-four-year-old biochemist at a medical school in the southern United States, he'd always been healthy. Right now, he was focused on completing a major research proposal. Omar finished his coffee and walked to a conference room near his laboratory to meet with his colleague, a cardiologist, to review the current version of the proposal. The deadline was January 15, and Omar realized that he had only four months to prepare his submission.

He settled into a chair, adjusted his wire-rimmed glasses, and spread out the pages of the proposal on the table in front of his colleague. "I don't know if it's just the light here," the cardiologist said, "but you look like you might be jaundiced."

Omar was surprised. He'd never had any problems with his liver.

"It's probably nothing," the doctor continued, "but you should get it checked out."

Omar didn't have a primary care doctor. He'd been meaning to select one after his physician had retired, but he hadn't gotten around to it.

"Why don't you call my internist," the cardiologist offered. "I'll let his office know that you'll be contacting them."

After the meeting, Omar looked in the mirror but didn't see any change in his eyes. He called the internist's office. The secretary told him that the doctor wanted him to stop by for blood tests so the results would be back in time for his appointment.

"In retrospect, I had been feeling tired for a while," Omar told us. "But I thought it was just because of my busy schedule. I had been staying up late working on the research proposal, and then I had to change time zones after a trip to Europe."

Omar picked up his son from a music lesson, and as soon as they returned home, he asked his wife, Ayesha, who taught linguistics at a local college, to look at his eyes. "She didn't see anything abnormal," he recounted. "Neither of us could really tell whether there was anything wrong."

A few days later, Omar went to see the internist. He greeted Omar warmly and then said, "I've heard from our mutual friend that your research is very cutting-edge."

Omar had been a precocious student, at the top of his class through high school and college. He came to the United States for his PhD in biochemistry and stayed for postdoctoral training, ultimately taking a position on the faculty at the medical school. Ayesha had been raised in the same town as Omar, and after finishing her degree in linguistics, they married and she moved to the United States to be with him. Many of Omar's relatives had since followed them to the United States.

"Your blood tests are back," the doctor said as he turned the computer screen on his desk so that Omar could see it. All of the test results were lit up in red. Omar's bilirubin, the yellow pigment that is normally passed through the liver and excreted in the stool, was elevated at 2.7, just at the level where jaundice can be detected. His transaminases, enzymes that reflect the health of the liver, were also abnormal, in the 200s. "But what was really frightening were my blood counts, my CBC," Omar told us. The doctor said he had "pancytopenia," meaning a low red cell blood count, reduced white blood cells, and a serious reduction in his platelet count.

The internist examined Omar and told him that he could feel the tip of his spleen below his left ribs, indicating that it was enlarged, but the liver was not enlarged or tender. The doctor ordered more blood tests and several days later called back and informed Omar that he had hepatitis B.

Hepatitis B is one of the most common viral liver infections in the world. It is particularly prevalent in Asia and the Middle East but also widespread in Europe and the Americas. Omar's son had been vaccinated against hepatitis B as part of the routine immunizations now given to children in the United States. "In my home country," Omar told us, "no one paid much attention to hepatitis B, and we were not vaccinated against it."

The hepatitis B virus was identified by Dr. Baruch Blumberg while he was studying the blood of Australian aboriginal peoples and was initially termed "Australia antigen." Blumberg won the Nobel Prize for this work in 1976. Routine vaccination of American children for hepatitis B began in 1991. More recently, drugs known as nucleoside analogues have been developed to treat hepatitis B infection. This new class of medications grew out of research on AIDS, where related drugs were found to potently block HIV. Although nucleoside analogues can have significant side effects, their use against AIDS and later hepatitis B infection has revolutionized treatment of these serious maladies. Omar was started on a drug called entecavir and was told that if it didn't work, there were similar medications that he could try, as well as experimental therapies. But these other treatments proved unnecessary; entecavir controlled the virus.

Despite this success, Omar's liver function tests worsened over the next two months. Scans of his liver and a biopsy showed cirrhosis, extensive scarring of the tissue from years of undetected hepatitis B infection. This was why the internist hadn't felt an enlarged liver when he examined Omar. Still, it wasn't clear why his blood tests didn't improve. "I felt good and was working full-time," Omar told us. "But my laboratory tests kept getting worse and worse." An extensive evaluation was undertaken to investigate why Omar's liver function was deteriorating. He was tested for parasites common in the Middle East that can affect the liver, queried about toxic solvents in his lab that might damage that organ, and screened for inherited disorders like

Wilson's disease that might cause cirrhosis in adult life. But no cause other than hepatitis B was found. His doctors kept waiting and hoping that things would improve. But they didn't.

"We need to start thinking about liver transplantation," the liver specialist at the medical center told Omar and Ayesha. "It's not definite that you'll need a transplant, but your liver is slowly deteriorating, and the treatment for the virus doesn't seem to be stopping that."

Omar and Ayesha were shocked to hear this. "Neither of us ever imagined a transplant," Omar said. "But the specialist told us that we'd have six to twelve months before the decision about transplant needed to be made. It wasn't a decision we had to make immediately. And that gave us a sense of relief."

Modern technology can support, at least temporarily, organs like the lungs with a ventilator, the heart with a bypass apparatus, and the kidneys with dialysis. The liver cannot be supported by a machine, but this vital organ can be transplanted. Dr. Joseph Murray of the Brigham and Women's Hospital in Boston pioneered organ transplantation. In 1954, he proved the long-term feasibility of the operation by beginning with identical twins. One healthy twin was able to donate his kidney to his ailing brother without concern about rejection, since they were genetically identical. This success spurred further research on how to overcome genetic barriers to transplanting the kidney, with refinements in selecting the organ not only from living donors but from cadavers.

Since Murray's achievement, which led to a Nobel Prize, the field of organ transplantation has expanded to include not only the kidney, but also the liver, heart, lungs, pancreas, and intestine. Each advance was enabled by progress in surgical technique and the development of new drugs that temper the recipient's immune system and reduce the chance that his or her body will reject the donated organ. Despite its considerable risks, transplantation can restore a very sick patient to a healthy life.

Although there has been much progress, transplantation is still fraught with uncertainty. Because donor organs are in such short supply, patients must be seriously ill to even be eligible for a liver transplant. Then a suitable liver must be obtained immediately after a donor's death, and the organ must be functioning and compatible with the recipient. The surgery itself is complex and demanding. The drugs that prevent rejection of the transplanted liver can have serious side effects, including putting the patient at risk for fatal infections or damaging the kidneys and lungs.

By the time a patient is poised to receive a new liver, he may not be capable of making choices for himself because his failing liver has caused confusion or even coma. Then it falls to family members or other surrogates to make decisions for him, as the doctors assess whether the intensive, uncertain, and extraordinarily expensive procedure of liver transplantation would be futile or lifesaving.

A month later, when Omar went in for a follow-up appointment with the liver specialist, his blood tests were much worse. He was planning two trips, one to the West Coast in December and one to Japan in January to attend scientific meetings. But the specialist insisted he cancel the trips. "We need to keep you close by. Your MELD score has reached the level where our transplant surgeon should evaluate you now."

MELD, short for "model for end-stage liver disease," is a calculation based on the patient's level of bilirubin, which indicates liver function; creatinine, which indicates kidney function; and a clotting test, which reflects the liver's ability to produce the proteins that make blood coagulate. A patient's MELD score is highly predictive of his or her chance of dying from advanced liver disease in the next twelve weeks. For that reason, liver transplantation centers use this score to determine which patients will get priority on waiting lists for donor organs. A patient's rank on a waiting list could have profound implications for survival. There are about seventeen thousand candidates slated for liver transplantation in the United States, but only five thousand transplants are performed each year. Many people die while waiting for a liver.

"When I saw the surgeon who directed the transplantation program—he was clearly very experienced—he told me, 'You know, at this point there is no way except transplantation.' That's when I started thinking really seriously about what I'm going to do. Where am I going to do the transplant? Which surgeon?" The more Omar read about liver transplantation, the more he saw how complex the procedure was, in part because it demanded very specific techniques with regard to harvesting the donated organ, transporting it to the recipient's medical center, and then transplanting successfully. Beyond the operation were choices the doctors would make that required highly specialized knowledge about which treatments to prevent the recipient's immune system from rejecting the foreign liver and how to combat infections not only from typical microbes like bacteria, but from so-called opportunistic pathogens like fungi and viruses that take root in tissues because of the patient's reduced immune defense.

Omar realized that regardless of how much research he did about liver transplantation, he and Ayesha would have to rely on his doctors to make critical decisions about his treatment. These decisions would involve not only technical aspects of the transplant, but how much to do should life-threatening complications occur.

Most centers begin listing patients for liver transplant when their MELD score reaches 10 or higher. But the MELD score at which a patient will actually receive a liver varies by region and medical center. A study done in 2007 by liver transplant researchers at the University of Pittsburgh, one of the major hospitals in the country performing this procedure, found that those centers with a high volume of transplants, one hundred or more per year, tend to transplant patients with lower MELD scores and have shorter waiting times than transplant centers that perform the procedure on smaller numbers of patients. The reasons for these differences weren't clear. The researchers speculated that high-volume centers might be willing to use organs that had been turned down by other transplant teams, shortening the waiting time. They also theorized that smaller centers that do fewer transplants might have personnel shortages for performing the procedure urgently, which might lengthen the waiting time for patients.

Omar learned that, indeed, different medical centers had different waiting times for patients in need of a liver transplant. He told us that he was also looking for data on the success rates of different surgical teams. "You know, I'm a scientist, I have a background in numbers. I realized that you can't just look at the reported outcomes alone. If there is a center that takes a lot of high-risk patients who have very high MELD scores and transplants them, then you expect that their figures might be worse than the success rate at a very conservative center which doesn't take high-risk patients, only good candidates with lower MELD scores."

Omar was still working full-time in his lab, trying to finish several experiments to be included in his grant proposal, which was due in just a few weeks. Shortly after noon, he closed his computer and went to grab a sandwich in the cafeteria. Waiting in line, he saw the surgeon who had evaluated him for transplantation. They nodded to each other, and then the surgeon walked with Omar to an empty table at the far end of the room.

"We'll be with you, no matter what you decide," the surgeon assured him. "If you choose to go with another center, we understand. But if you stay with us, I promise you, we are committed to you and to every one of the people we care for."

"Thank you," Omar said. "I understand."

As Omar continued his research, the choices before him seemed only to multiply. He learned about the "living donor" liver transplant, a procedure begun in 1998 that has become increasingly used because of the scarcity of livers from deceased donors. In this procedure, a healthy person matched for blood type has part of his liver removed; the excised part of the organ is then transplanted into the recipient. There are small but significant risks to the donor, but in most cases the procedure is safe. Very rarely, complications have resulted in the donor's death. Omar's medical center didn't perform living donor liver transplantation, so he contacted another medical center where these transplants were done.

A senior surgeon there reviewed Omar's medical records, then they spoke by phone. "You have a very high MELD score," the surgeon said. "And we really don't like to do living donor transplants with scores this high. But the notes say that you're still working." Omar replied that indeed he was and that everyone who knew him was surprised that he felt as good as he did and could keep working despite the deteriorating liver and kidney function tests. "In that case, living donor transplantation may be an option for you if you have a match," the surgeon concluded.

Omar was aware of the risks to the donor who gave part of his or her liver: "I initially refused to have anybody from my family be a donor. It's a risky surgery. I didn't want to drag anybody down with me." Ayesha pleaded with him to let her donate part of her liver if she was a good match. But he refused. "At least our son should have one of us around." Many of Omar's relatives insisted they be tested as potential donors. Two of them were genetically compatible, and each volunteered. But their subsequent medical evaluations revealed that one, who was a heavy smoker, had heart disease, and the other had an inherited abnormality in a clotting protein, making the risk of bleeding from major surgery very high.

"So I realized my transplant options were limited," Omar told us. "And I began to follow the waiting lists at different medical centers, and track data about which states had the most available organs. I wondered whether I should move to a different state; it might save my life."

Working late one Sunday night to finish his grant proposal, Omar developed chills and a high fever. He was admitted to the hospital and found to have an infected cut on his foot that had allowed bacteria into his bloodstream. He stayed in the hospital for a week to receive antibiotics. Ayesha arranged for a neighbor to look after their son and spent every evening at Omar's bedside. The transplantation team, including the senior surgeon, saw him every day during this hospitalization. Omar was impressed by how thorough and attentive they were and decided that he would have his transplant done with this team.

Based on his research, Omar knew it was likely he wouldn't be able to make decisions himself through the course of transplant. When patients lose the ability to make medical decisions, the surrogate decision maker may be called on to make what is termed a "substituted judgment," identifying the decision that the patient would have made if he'd been able to do so. The concept of substituted judgment was established in 1976 with the famous court case of Karen Ann Quinlan. The New Jersey Supreme Court designated her father as the surrogate decision maker since she was in a persistent vegetative state; the charge from the judge was to make a health care decision for her in a way that reflected how she would have made that decision herself if she was able.

Since then, substituted judgment has been the guiding framework for surrogate decision making in bioethics and law, because it protects the principle of patient autonomy. However, considerable research indicates that even when surrogates have had prior discussions with a patient about his or her preferences or have the patient's advance directive in writing, they often fail to choose the option that corresponds to the patient's wishes. In an analysis of more than a dozen studies constituting nearly twenty-six hundred surrogate-patient pairs presented with hypothetical scenarios that required them to make choices about treatment, the surrogate failed to correctly predict the patient's preferences a third of the time. Further complicating the surrogates' task is the fact that patients' preferences aren't fixed, so what the patient would actually choose in the future is hard to predict.

Dr. Alexia M. Torke, a prominent researcher in geriatrics and medical ethics at the Regenstrief Institute and the Indiana University Center for Aging Research in Indianapolis, wrote about substituted judgment, "Since the theoretical framework for surrogate decision making was developed, research has shown that the concept of substituted judgment rests upon false assumptions and is unable to meet the standard goals of maintaining patient autonomy."

A second principle may be invoked when the patient can't make his or her own decisions: "beneficence." This principle dictates that doctors and other medical personnel have the obligation to act in the patient's own "best legitimate interests." While the principles of patient autonomy and beneficence may coincide, there are times when what a patient said she wanted in an advance directive or what family surrogates imagine she would want clashes with what the treating doctors believe is in her best interests. In such cases, the courts and the majority of ethicists have concluded that autonomy trumps beneficence.

Yet a study done by Dr. Torke and colleagues reveals that physicians often do not make the wishes of the patient or the surrogate their top priority when formulating decisions about care. In a survey of 281 physicians, although nearly three-quarters of doctors endorsed patient preferences as the most important ethical standard for surrogate decision making, only 30 percent said patient preference was the primary factor in their most recent real-world decision. While these doctors considered the principle of autonomy, they more frequently ranked as most important what they viewed was in the best interests of the patient—the principle of beneficence. Even when the patients had prepared advance directives or living wills, these doctors viewed patient preference as the key factor in their decisions less than half the time.

Torke offered several possible explanations for these findings. As we noted in the previous chapter, advance directives or prior conversations with the patient about care may not apply to the clinical situation at hand. In addition, although physicians are taught that autonomy should be given priority in patient and surrogate decision making, they may perceive that acting in the patient's best interests is at least equally important; many doctors feel a sense of duty to determine and promote the patient's best interests. Furthermore, Torke wondered whether physicians may make "global assessments" that include both best interests and patient preferences.

As the need for a transplant became ever more urgent, Ayesha pressed Omar to give her guidance about her role in treatment decisions, since she would be his surrogate.

"I want you to do anything that the doctors say is acceptable," Omar stated.

Ayesha promised she would.

Omar had developed a sense of trust and confidence in his transplantation team. He believed that this team of doctors and nurses would be focused on him, that his best interests were at the forefront of their thinking. Despite his extensive research into the technical aspects of liver transplantation, Omar had decided that for him, the principle of autonomy could be secondary to the principle of beneficence.

Other patients hold fast to the principle of autonomy, even when faced with highly specialized and complex treatments. Some contend that knowledge gained from expert opinions, the Internet, and books about the condition and its remedies can give them enough information to retain their autonomy rather than relying on their doctors' beneficence. Other patients may have experienced a misdiagnosis or medical mistake, an error in judgment on the part of doctors or nurses, an event that limited how much trust they could place in clinicians regardless of their reputation or character. Others feel that only a close family member or friend acting as a surrogate can truly imagine what their wishes would be under dire and rapidly changing circumstances.

Omar recovered from the infection and returned to work. But he found that he had no energy to review the data from experiments, no ability to focus on the final pages of the grant proposal. The cardiologist who was collaborating with him agreed to finish writing the proposal on his own.

A week later, Omar again developed a fever and then pain in his abdomen. Ayesha took him to the emergency room, and he was found to have another infection. This time it was peritonitis, an infection in the fluid in his abdomen. As Omar dozed off in the ER, the attending physician spoke to Ayesha. "His liver is deteriorating," he said, showing her the printout of Omar's blood tests. "And his kidneys are shutting down."

Ayesha's dark brown eyes welled with tears.

"We need to get him to the ICU. He is seriously, seriously ill."

Ayesha told us, "We had been so hopeful, and expected that we would have six to twelve months to arrange everything." Now, that time had telescoped to what might be a matter of weeks or even days.

By morning, Omar was comatose. The ICU doctors were infusing antibiotics and gauging the amount of intravenous fluid to give since his kidneys were not producing urine. Omar's abdomen became more swollen and tense as the infection spread. Two days later, the news got worse. Omar was found to have not only a bacterial infection in his abdomen and bloodstream, but also a fungus. Fungal infections are especially hard to eradicate, and the antibiotics used to treat them, which are metabolized in the liver, are quite toxic, particularly to the kidneys. On the fourth day in the ICU, Omar began to bleed internally, a frequent complication of severe liver disease. The medical team transfused him and performed a procedure to try to seal off the bleeding vessels.

"I never expected things to happen that fast," Ayesha told us. "But everything was changing within hours. He was in really bad condition, and it was too difficult for him to breathe on his own. So he had to be put on a ventilator." The ICU doctors gave her papers to sign first to put him on a ventilator and then to start dialysis since his kidneys were failing.

"I just signed each paper," Ayesha told us. She shared Omar's trust and confidence in the transplant team and felt that the doctors were acting in his best interests. In this instance, there was no clash between autonomy and beneficence.

Not every surrogate is fortunate enough to know the doctors caring for a loved one. People incapacitated after a major car accident, a massive heart attack, or a stroke are rushed to the hospital, where their family members may be meeting the doctors for the first time. In such cases, when you don't know the doctor and the doctor doesn't know you or your loved one, it can be difficult to trust that he or she understands what the patient's "best interests" are. This can result in an adversarial relationship between physician and surrogate. Surrogates may wonder, Are the doctors jumping to conclusions about my loved one's prognosis? Are the hospital and doctors being pressured by insurers to limit costly care? If the loved one is elderly, do the doctors have an "ageist" bias; are they leery of providing intensive treatments for older people?

Some researchers have suggested that surrogates should share the narrative of the person's life with the physicians. By doing so, the family can help the doctor realize that beyond the catheters, tubes, monitors, and machines that surround the incapacitated patient, there is a person. Dr. Alexia Torke of Indiana University observes that this focus on the patient's life story "can build a common purpose and understanding among surrogates and health care providers. It retains the psychological advantage in turning attention from the needs and wishes of the patient's loved ones to those of the patient, but maintains the realistic perspective of what we can know about the patient."

When considering the patient's life story, both surrogates and physicians may find helpful the framework that we've already outlined for identifying one's own preferences, how they arose, and what has shaped them: the attitudes and values of the family, prior medical experiences, encounters with others who may have faced similar conditions and made choices. Of course, there may be gaps in this second-hand narrative because only the patient could tell the full story. But even parts of the narrative might help surrogates and physicians better understand the patient's preferences and mind-set.

W
ith each day, Omar's MELD score rose until he reached a level where death was predicted to be likely and soon. "If there's someone you need to tell about Omar's condition," the ICU doctor said, "I think now is the time to call. We don't know how much longer he will live."

Ayesha sat frozen for a long moment. Until then, she hadn't re-ally absorbed the severity of his condition. "At that point, it started really hitting me," she told us. Ayesha called one of Omar's brothers who was a physician. He said that he would come as soon as he could. "But he told me that I was the one who had to make decisions," Ayesha said. "And that was really difficult for me. Because the burden was entirely on me."

Each day Ayesha spent long hours in the waiting room, looking for what she termed a "streak of hope" that Omar would improve and a liver would become available. "Every hour the doctors had to treat one problem after another, doing all sorts of things, changing intravenous lines, tubes, the dialysis, trying to get the infection under control."

After two weeks in the ICU, he was still in a coma, and his kidneys produced hardly any urine. Although the bleeding had stopped and the infection was under control, Ayesha knew that his condition was dire. "At first they told me that because Omar was young and strong, they wanted to wait to make sure they got a good liver. Then, the trans-plant surgeon came by to speak with me. 'So far, we haven't been able to get a liver,' he said. 'If one becomes available, even if it's infected with hepatitis C, we would need to transplant it because we've reached a point where we don't know if he will survive one more day.'"

Ayesha asked him, "But what does that mean to give Omar a diseased liver?"

"It could be lifesaving," the surgeon said. "It doesn't mean that he would be sick immediately, but he would need to be treated for that virus, which isn't simple, and the donated liver could deteriorate. He might have to be transplanted a second time."

The doctor paused, then added, "We need to know whether you would agree that we should go ahead under those circumstances."

Ayesha was stunned. "I have to think about it," she replied after a moment.

Here, decision making shifted back from the doctors to Ayesha as the surrogate.

Besides autonomy and beneficence, ethicists and lawyers have identified another principle that can apply to medical decisions: nonmaleficence. Put simply, this means not inflicting harm. The dictum "First do no harm," attributed to Hippocrates, is a foundational tenet of Western medicine and dates back millennia. The principle can be invoked when patients or surrogates assert their autonomy and request treatments that the doctor believes have little or no benefit and might well be harmful. In such settings, ethicists and lawyers contend that the physician can refuse to participate in practices he or she judges to be dangerous to the patient.

The principle of nonmaleficence applied to the choice that Ayesha was facing. To accept a liver infected with hepatitis C might be giving Omar a new and serious disease. On the other hand, the diseased organ could save his life. Here, the doctors were navigating between beneficence and nonmaleficence, because transplanting a diseased liver had elements of both. So the physicians returned to the principle of autonomy—they wanted Omar's surrogate to decide.

That evening, Ayesha called one of Omar's close friends, a gastroenterologist. "He told me just to say yes to the hepatitis C liver," she recounted. "I should take anything that comes up. He explained that the surgeon would not propose this if Omar was not in extreme danger."

Ayesha spent the rest of the night anticipating regret, debating in her mind the answer she would give the surgeon. "I was worried that I would end up giving Omar another disease," she told us. "Treatment for hepatitis C would be difficult, and then he might need another transplant. It made me feel guilty. But I would have felt guiltier if I had said no." Ayesha told us, as day broke, that she spent more than an hour crying and then called the surgeon to give her permission. "This was lifesaving treatment—I knew I had to say yes."

Two more days passed, and, as Ayesha told us, Omar was "hanging by a thread." She recalled that he had contacted another medical center where living donor transplants were done, and in desperation she called the director of that program. "I wanted to make sure that I'd done everything. I said what if I moved him over there? But the doctor at the other medical center said that Omar was too sick to be transferred, and that once someone was on a ventilator, they didn't do a living donor transplant."

Omar's surgeon understood that Ayesha wanted her husband to live "at all costs." At this point, for Ayesha, there was no loss aversion, no anticipated regret, no contemplating the potential side effects of attempting to transplant someone with his severity of illness, no real forecasting of what Omar's life would be like should he survive. "There was no side effect that could be worse than the way he was at that time," she told us. Every trade-off paled before that reality. "I'm not very religious, but I have faith," Ayesha told us. She sat at Omar's bedside, praying and reading verses from the Koran on healing. "I knew that everything was being done that could be done, and everything else was in the hands of God."

One night in the ICU, she was leafing through a magazine and read an article about Chris Klug, an alpine snowboarder from Aspen, Colorado. In the early 1990s, on a routine physical exam, Klug was found to have a rare liver disease called primary sclerosing cholangitis. At the time, he was at peak athletic fitness, successfully competing at the highest level with no symptoms at all. For years, Klug felt good, although his liver function tests continued to deteriorate. Then he got sick, and his MELD score rose. He was on the waiting list for three months before he received a donor liver. The transplant was successful, and seven weeks after the surgery he was back on the slopes training. In 2002, he took the bronze medal at the Salt Lake City Olympics. "To win a medal after a liver transplant," Ayesha told us, showed her that "despite how sick someone might be, he might return to a vigorous life."

This anecdote buoyed Ayesha up. Availability became a source of hope, helping her cope with the harsh reality of Omar's condition. On a strictly clinical level, Chris Klug's story wasn't comparable to Omar's: Klug's type of liver disease was quite different, and he hadn't been nearly as close to death as Omar, who had bacterial and fungal bloodstream infections, kidney failure, internal bleeding, and coma. But reading this vignette helped Ayesha hold on to hope for Omar.

Late in the afternoon of January 17, the surgeon spoke with Ayesha.

"We're not sure he'll live another day," he said.

Ayesha nodded.

She went home late that evening, called Omar's brother, and told him what the surgeon had said. She put her son to bed and said her prayers before falling asleep.

At one a.m., the telephone rang and woke her up.

"We can get a liver from out of state," the surgeon said. "Two other centers have passed on it because it came from an older person who had cancer and had chemotherapy. We aren't sure, but this person also may have been exposed to hepatitis C."

Ayesha took a moment to ponder what the surgeon saying. "You said Omar might die today."

"That's true. Of course, no one can ever say precisely when someone will die," the surgeon replied. "But he is at the very edge."

"I want you to go ahead," Ayesha said.

We spoke with Omar and Ayesha about a year and a half after the transplant. He had spent two months in rehabilitation and then several more months at home to regain his strength with physical therapy. Now he was back at work full-time. "I feel great," he told us. "I take my medications to prevent rejection of the graft, my antiviral therapy to keep hepatitis B from recurring, and the liver is working well. I know that the liver came from an older patient who had been treated for cancer, and it was rejected by two other centers. I realize how desperate the surgeons had to be to use it. But thank God they did. That liver saved my life."

Things could have turned out very differently. Omar might not have survived the transplant despite the best efforts of his doctors. In fact, after Omar recovered, one of the residents told Ayesha that the transplant team hadn't expected him to live. One of the senior physicians in the ICU had told a colleague that she'd never seen anyone that sick survive. Consider also that even if Omar survived, he may have been left severely debilitated, paralyzed, unable to speak, or even in a vegetative state.

These kinds of unknowns apply to many of the patients who

populate our ICUs. Patients with catastrophic illnesses typically require "heroic measures." These may include prolonged respiratory support on a ventilator, renal dialysis, catheters threaded into the chambers of their hearts, and a host of other invasive and risky interventions that offer no guarantee the patient will survive. And if he survives, in what condition?

Several studies have examined how accurately physicians predict the trajectory of disease in sick patients. Research done among patients in the ICU found that doctors are generally correct in giving a prognosis for moderately ill patients, but they aren't very good at predicting the course of the sickest patients. In one study conducted in Paris, physicians erred on both sides—too optimistic and too pessimistic.

For that reason, critical care physicians have devised metrics to indicate when further treating severely ill patients would be "futile." The mortality probability model (MPM-II) estimates the likelihood of death in the hospital. The model has been applied in studies of decision making about whether to admit a patient to the ICU and also to predict the prognosis after one day of intensive treatment there. Researchers from a consortium of hospitals in Massachusetts evaluated the MPM-II and concluded that "no system has been perfected to the point where decisions regarding an individual patient can be based on the estimated probabilities produced. This is especially true when considering denying a patient admission to the ICU on the basis of the estimated probability."

The APACHE II score* is another calculation based on organ function that's frequently used to predict the probability of life or death in very sick patients. A study done at Guy's Hospital in London

---

* Acute physiology and chronic health evaluation (APACHE II) score.

applied this metric each day to thirty-six hundred patients in the intensive care unit. The researchers concluded that the APACHE II calculation was imperfect: One of twenty patients predicted to die actually lived, and most of those who survived had a good quality of life. Using such a system to decide when to withdraw treatment therefore might cost the life of some people who would otherwise survive with a reasonable quality of life. The researchers commented that the degree of predictive error that is generally "acceptable" reflects the value placed upon an individual human life in a particular culture or society. For that reason, they suggested that the APACHE II score should not "necessitate" withdrawing treatment, but rather "focus the attention" of the doctor and the patient's surrogate on discussing "in a more informed fashion" the nature of the condition. They concluded that treatment should be withdrawn only if "this was in the patient's best interests." Because a formula for futility seemed impossible to devise, the authors invoked the principle of beneficence, the "best interests" of the patient.

The decision to stop treating a patient is one of the most agonizing in medicine. Doctors don't give up on many of the sickest patients for the sake of the few like Omar who will survive catastrophic illness and return to life.

Boris Veysman, a senior emergency care physician at the University of Medicine & Dentistry of New Jersey, wrote in 2010 in the journal *Health Affairs* of his own changing attitude about the meaning of futility: "In my role as a doctor, I've met countless disabled, disfigured, machine-supported people who enjoy living and wish to continue doing so as long as possible. I've met intensive care survivors who lead full, productive lives, often with few or no memories of their ordeals and heroic procedures because their sedation was done correctly. . . .

"Life is precious and irreplaceable. Even severe incurable illness can often be temporarily fixed, moderated, or controlled, and most discomfort can be made tolerable or even pleasant with simple drugs. In chess, to resign is to give up the game with pieces and options remaining. My version of DNR is 'Do Not Resign.' Don't give up on me if I can still think, communicate, create, and enjoy life. When taking care of me, take care of yourself as well, to make sure you don't burn out by the time I need your optimism the most.

"It's so easy to let someone die, but it takes effort, determination, and stamina to help someone stay and feel alive."

Ayesha shared this view. "Whatever might be lifesaving," she told us, "I wanted for Omar. So long as the doctors believed there was even a small chance to save his life, it was worth trying. Everything else was secondary."

Of course, such care is expensive. Some health care economists and policy planners seek a monetary cutoff that will clearly dictate whether to start or continue costly treatments. But Michael K. Gusmano and Daniel Callahan of the Hastings Center in New York, who have extensively studied the ethics of medical economics, point out in a 2011 *Annals of Internal Medicine* article, "What may be a good value for money for a sick person may not be good value for other members of society." So where do you draw the line? Gusmano and Callahan continue, "Formal economic evaluations try to address this issue by adopting explicit standards that specify and place limits on the economic value of health benefits. Yet . . . setting the standard is crucial and problematic."

The standard that has been most widely proposed is the quality-adjusted life year (QALY). A QALY is a measure of one year of added life adjusted up or down for the quality of life during that year. In the United Kingdom, the National Institute for Health and Clinical Excellence (NICE) relies on the QALY in determining whether a new treatment will be approved for general use. Although NICE does not have an explicit monetary cutoff, it tends to use a cost-per-QALY amount between £20,000 (about $30,000) and £30,000 (about $42,000) in order to approve a new drug or device.

Although one year of life is an objective measure, critics of QALYs have pointed out that the quality of life for any individual during that year is clearly subjective and can't be assessed accurately by using any currently available method. Paul Dolan, a professor of economics at Imperial College London, contends that the approach NICE uses to formulate QALYs is flawed. Healthy people are asked to generate numbers on clinical conditions using time trade-off or standard gamble methods that we described in chapter 5. Dolan criticizes this strategy since healthy people, as we have previously discussed, can't accurately imagine life with a medical condition they have never experienced. The Nobel laureate Daniel Kahneman likened QALY measurements to the attempts by nineteenth-century physicists to measure the viscosity of the "ether" in the universe, an ether that did not exist. Despite such serious criticisms, numerous experts in the public and private sectors are now proposing QALYs to guide expenditures as part of American health care reform.

Surrogates find guidance in the ethical principles of autonomy, beneficence, and nonmaleficence. We believe that further insight may be gained by considering the vocabulary that reflects the mind-sets of the many patients we spoke with: believers and doubters; maximalists and minimalists; a naturalism orientation or a technology orientation.

For example, Dr. Veysman is a believer, a maximalist, with a technology orientation; he believes that modern medicine can succeed even against long odds. Omar and his doctors were of the same mind-set; they were also maximalists and believers in science and technology; they didn't view as futile the many intensive measures needed to keep Omar alive before and through his liver transplant. Ayesha as the surrogate "representing Omar" also adopted this mind-set. Other incapacitated patients may have taken a different approach to their health during their lives, as doubters or minimalists or with a naturalism orientation.

By considering the patient's life story, surrogates and physicians can separate their own mind-sets from the patient's. This way, they can better choose for the patient who can't decide for himself.

Conclusion

*Every patient carries her or
his own doctor inside.*

—ALBERT SCHWEITZER

I f medicine were an exact science, like mathematics, there would be
one correct answer for each problem. Your preferences about treatment would be irrelevant to what is "right." But medicine is an
uncertain science.

Studies and statistics can tell us that one or two in a group of one
hundred women like Susan Powell with high cholesterol will have a
heart attack. But which ones? Similarly, we can't identify with certainty the one or two women out of three hundred who will benefit
by taking a statin drug. Even genetic information like BRCA testing
provides only an estimate of cancer risk. No one can say which women
will develop breast cancer and when. Nor can we say with certainty
what impact atrial fibrillation or prostate cancer or any other condi-

tion will have on an individual's life or how someone will experience the side effects from a particular treatment. Each of us is unique in the interplay of genetic makeup and environment. The path to maintaining or regaining health is not the same for everyone.

Choices made in this gray zone are frequently not simple or obvious. For that reason, medicine involves nuanced and personalized decision making by both the patient and the doctor.

This essential truth is often overlooked by experts who seek to standardize treatments rather than customize them to the individual. Although presented as scientific, formulas that reduce the experience of illness to numbers are flawed and artificial. Yet insurers and government officials are pressuring physicians and hospitals to standardize care using such formulas. Policy planners and even some doctors have declared that the art of medicine is passé, that care should be delivered in an industrialized fashion with doctors and nurses following operating manuals. They contend that doctors and patients can't be relied upon to decide what is best. While they insist that their aim is "patient-centered care," in fact it is "system-centered care."

Recently, we heard from a colleague at another hospital that an administrator sits in the clinic and times how long it takes for a patient to move from the waiting room to the examining room and how many minutes are spent with the doctor. This is being done to improve "efficiency." But people need time to explore the roots of their preferences and to consider whether their thinking is truly in their best interests. Such deep deliberation with a doctor is not "efficient," it does not fit into a vision of the clinic and hospital as assembly lines.

Your preferences about treatment do matter. They provide a foundation so that you can choose the right treatment, the one that fits your values and way of living. Understanding your preferences begins with reflecting on your mind-set.

Studies show that some 60 percent of people in the United States pursue so-called alternative or natural therapies. This indicates a naturalism orientation, the notion that the body can often heal itself if given the proper environment, harnessing the mind-body connection and supplementing with herbs, vitamins, and other natural products. On the opposite end of this spectrum is the technology orientation, the belief that cutting-edge research yielding new medications and innovative procedures holds the answers.

Each of us also falls somewhere along a second spectrum, depending on whether we want maximal or minimal treatment. Some people are proudly proactive about their health, believing that more is usually better. Even in the absence of definitive clinical data, some patients and indeed some physicians believe that they will be healthier and live longer by tightly controlling their blood pressure or dramatically reducing their "bad" LDL cholesterol or achieving a body mass index below recommended levels; they are intent on being "ahead of the curve." In contrast, those with a minimalist mind-set aim to avoid treatment if at all possible; and if that is not possible, they try to use the fewest medications at the lowest possible doses or to select the most conservative surgery or procedure. Minimalists hold to the notion that "less is more," that risks and unintended consequences may overshadow apparent benefits.

Then there are believers and doubters. Believers approach their options with the sense that there is a successful solution for their problem somewhere. They generally have a well-defined orientation. Doubters approach all treatment options with profound skepticism. They are deeply risk-averse, acutely aware of the potential side effects and limitations of drugs and procedures. They question how much benefit a therapy really offers them and whether there might be deleterious consequences.

A believer can have a strong naturalism orientation, trusting in the healing power of nature and shunning high-tech interventions.

Or a believer can have a technology orientation, relying on the promise of modern medicine. A believer who is a maximalist feels that more treatment is the best approach and doing less is shortsighted, whereas a believer who is a minimalist is certain of the opposite strategy. For example, one of our friends is a believer, a maximalist with a strong naturalism orientation; his cabinets and refrigerator are filled with nutritional supplements, he has regular acupuncture treatments to "stay healthy," and he consults a homeopathic practitioner for any illnesses. Another friend, also a believer with a strong naturalism orientation, is a minimalist. She takes no supplements on a regular basis, but when treatment seems necessary, she prefers herbal remedies in the smallest amounts. Similarly, those believers with a technology orientation may be maximalists or minimalists.

Doubters are typically minimalists. They apply their skepticism without consideration to the origins of a therapy, whether it be prescribed medications or herbal supplements. Some people are doubters at the outset, drawing on the attitudes of their upbringing, while others arrive at this mind-set through hard experience after an incorrect diagnosis or a treatment that falls short of expectations.

Being a doubter is uncomfortable, because it results in intense decisional conflict. While doubt can prevent you from making an impulsive choice, it can also be paralyzing. In the end, when we are ill, we all want to believe that there is a treatment worth taking.

After you consider your mind-set with regard to these categories, it is valuable to go through a deliberate process to become informed and to better understand the often hidden influences that can sway your thinking and distort your judgment.

The Institute of Medicine of the National Academy of Sciences places "informed patient choice" at the "pinnacle of quality medical care." But this begs the question: What does it really mean to be informed? It means knowing the numbers about a particular medication or procedure, its likely benefits and side effects, but it also means being alert to how the presentation of these numbers can confuse or mislead you.

Stating that 35 percent of people with a serious illness are cured by a certain treatment has a hopeful resonance, while stating that 65 percent of people die despite that therapy has a pessimistic sound. But both statements are factually correct and describe the same data. For that reason, it is always valuable to "flip the frame" in your mind, to view information in both its positive and its negative forms.

Framing can be even more subtle, using words instead of numbers. For example, stating that a drug works "in the majority of patients" sounds quite different from specifying that 51 percent of people responded to the treatment, yet both are accurate. It is important to understand the numbers behind the words.

Finally, to most clearly understand the true benefit of a treatment, try to learn the "number needed to treat," how many people with a condition similar to yours need to receive a therapy in order to improve or cure one person. Similarly, the "number needed to harm," how many people typically must receive the treatment in order for one to suffer a side effect, more clearly reveals the risk of a therapy. Decision aids often contain these numbers, or your physician may give them to you. The number needed to treat contributed to Susan Powell's decision not to take a statin drug. She discovered how the expected benefit of the drug applied to her as an individual and valued that result in light of her particular mind-set: a doubter and minimalist. Of course, for another person like Michelle Byrd, a believer and maximalist with a technology orientation, the same number needed to treat could reinforce her aim to be proactive, to do everything possible to avoid future illness.

It is vital when making a treatment choice that you remain alert to cognitive pitfalls beyond framing of numbers. By unmasking these hidden influences, you can gain a greater sense of confidence that your decision process was sound. For example, research from psychology shows that all of us generally experience loss more profoundly than gain. This aversion to loss may cause you to give undue weight to possible side effects compared with expected benefits.

Another powerful influence on thinking is the "focusing illusion." In trying to forecast the future, all of us tend to focus on a particular aspect of our lives that would be negatively affected by a proposed treatment. This then becomes the overriding element in decision making. The focusing illusion neglects our extraordinary capacity to adapt, to enjoy life with less than "perfect" health. Imagining life with a colostomy, after a mastectomy, or following prostate surgery can all be skewed by the focusing illusion. We cannot see how the remaining parts of our lives expand to fill the gaps created by the illness and its treatment.

Seeing how those gaps may be filled can come from learning about the experiences of others with the same condition. This powerful influence of stories on thinking is termed "availability." If a relative or friend was able to adapt successfully following a therapy, this may help you to see your own future with a wider focus. On the other hand, if your father or sister or a close friend had a severe side effect from a drug or operation, you will be unlikely to choose as they did. Even if you don't personally know someone who has benefited or been hurt by a particular treatment, the news media and Internet provide countless tales and testimonials that can become the basis for "availability bias." It is impossible to dismiss the power of availability. For many people, it is the primary factor in determining their preferences.

But availability can also work to your detriment. It can cause you to distort the reality of what you face. To avoid this, it is best to integrate stories into the larger body of information, meaning the numbers about risk and benefit, particularly the number needed to treat and the number needed to harm.

As you go through this deliberate process of analyzing information, attentive to cognitive pitfalls, also consider how much autonomy or control you want in decision making. Some of the people we interviewed went to great lengths to exert control over every aspect of their medical care. Others did not. Just as there is no "one size fits all" in treatment, there is not a single choice about how much control you should want. Rather, try to find your starting place on the spectrum of autonomy, and then, as your trust and confidence in your doctors is confirmed or lost, consider again if that position makes sense.

We are often asked who is the "best doctor" to treat a particular condition. One criterion is a physician's knowledge about your condition and its treatments, his or her command of the scientific data, so-called evidence-based medicine. But we believe the best doctors go one step further and practice "judgment-based medicine," meaning they consider available evidence and then assess how it applies to the individual patient.

Some patients seek physicians who have a mind-set like their own: a maximalist patient may prefer a maximalist doctor, while a minimalist patient may want a doctor with that approach. Yet Dr. Jacques Carter cares for Susan Powell and Michelle Byrd and Alex Miller, each with a different mind-set. Although he doesn't agree with all their choices, he tries to understand the orientation and values of each, and he shows respect even when his preferences differ from theirs. While you don't want a doctor who superimposes his or her own preferences on you, you may not gain as much from a doctor who just rubber-stamps your decisions. A doctor who facilitates but also may challenge your decision process sometimes gives you more.

Writing this book changed us. It changed how we, as physicians, help our patients make decisions about treatment. Each day at work, as we speak with people facing different treatment options, we find ourselves using the terms that arose from this book: minimalists and maximalists; believers and doubters; naturalism or technology orientation. We find ourselves thinking more about autonomy and regret while helping patients make their decisions. As we introduced this vocabulary, patients have taken the words and concepts and expanded on them to better explain their point of view and mind-set. Writing this book also changed how we weigh options about our own health, defining and showing us the origins and evolution of our preferences.

Navigating a medical decision is a dynamic process. Your orientation and mind-set, the level of autonomy you desire, and the influences you are exposed to may change over the course of time. We hope that the insights provided in this book will help you to better understand your approach to health before entering the doctor's office or hospital, to clearly explain your thinking to your physician, and then to continue the decision-making process after you leave. Then you will be on the path to choosing the right treatment for the right reasons.

Acknowledgments

We are deeply grateful to the many patients and their family members who shared their stories with us, opening their hearts and minds. Our debt to each is beyond words. We have worked hard to capture the thoughts, feelings, and lessons they wished to communicate. Any shortcomings in substance or style are ours.

Our agent, Suzanne Gluck at William Morris Endeavour, was the catalyst for this project. Her belief that we could work together as a team, each one complementing the other, gave us the courage to begin and persist in writing this book. At each step in the process, her insights and constructive criticisms were invaluable.

Eamon Dolan was our editor at the Penguin Press. He shepherded us with a firm hand and wry sense of humor, pulling us back when we veered astray. Eamon relentlessly (and in the kindest possible way) pushed us to express our ideas on the page in a lucid and cogent manner. Any writer who works with him is fortunate, indeed. Ann Godoff applied her keen intellect and incomparable skills as a publisher to shape the book. Her vision and commitment mean so much to us. We are also deeply thankful to the other members of the Penguin Press who contributed their expertise: Sarah Hutson, Tracy Locke, Emily Graff, Katherine Griggs, Sona Vogel, and Darren Haggar.

Special thanks to Shelly Harrison for her talent in creating our author photographs.

As is clear from both the narratives and the endnotes, we drew from many disciplines, including psychology, cognitive science, economics, history, mathematics, and, of course, medicine. The scope of our inquiry called on the extraordinary efforts of an extraordinary person. That person is Youngsun Jung, and her diligence and intelligence in researching ideas, fact checking, and manuscript preparation are unparalleled.

We received support, encouragement, and suggestions from numerous friends and colleagues: Ron Ansin, Arthur Cohen, Tom Dyja, Nora Ephron, Myron Falchuk, Carol Greenlee, Rabbi William Hamilton, Susan Harrison, James Hennessey, Tony Hollenberg, Keith Johnson, Alex Joseph, Hercules Kyriazidis, Annik LaFarge, Emily Lazar, Anika Lucas, Norman Manea, Ted Marmor, Ben Mizell, Peter Moschensen, Stephen Nimer, Johanna Pallotta, Nick Pileggi, Thomas Ramsey; Dina, Michael, and Oudi Recanati; Frank Rich, Maria Rossano, Harold Rosen, Julie Sandorf, Stuart Schoffman, Shanti Serdy, Michael Share, Judy Shih, Jodi Silton, Chris Smith, Abe and Cindy Steinberger, Jeffrey Tepler, Sarah Elizabeth Button White, Jay Winik, Alex Witchel, and Ed Zwick. During the writing of the book, we met Rabbi Yitzchok Itkin and Rebbetzin Chanie Itkin. Their strength and wisdom inspired us, and we honor the memory of their beloved daughter, Chaya Mushka, ז״ל.

Our family is populated by believers and doubters, maximalists and minimalists, some with a naturalism orientation and others with a technology orientation. We thank them all for their opinions. Our children, Steve, Mike, and Emily, endured countless dinner discussions about this project (not always willingly). They did not hesitate to pass judgment on how we shaped our points and crafted our prose. We also received key input from our sibs, Meryl, Lori, Lenny, and Judy.

Acknowledgments

Over the past years, we honed our thinking and individual and joint writing skills through our work with Ryan DuBosar and Janet Colwell at the *ACP Internist*, Debbie Malina at the *New England Journal of Medicine*, David Remnick, Dorothy Wickenden, Henry Finder, Daniel Zalewski, and Andrea Thompson at the *New Yorker*, Robert Silvers at the *New York Review of Books*, Dorothy Rabinowitz and Robert Pollock at the *Wall Street Journal*, David Shipley at the *New York Times*, and Marty Peretz and Leon Wieseltier at the *New Republic*. We thank them all.

Notes

INTRODUCTION

1   A national survey of common medical decisions, made by adults forty and older in the United States, was conducted by researchers at the University of Michigan. The results indicate that over a two-year period, thirty-three million people considered medication for an elevated cholesterol level, twenty-seven million for high blood pressure, and sixteen million for depression; ten million people considered cataract surgery, seven million hip or knee replacement, and seven million an operation for low back pain. See: Brian J. Zikmund-Fisher et al., "The decision study: A nationwide survey of United States adults regarding 9 common medical decisions," *Medical Decision Making* 30 (2010), pp. S20–S34.

2   Atrial fibrillation, the abnormal heart rhythm that Dave Simon has, is increasingly frequent in both the United States and Europe. About 1 to 2 percent of the population suffers from the condition, and this figure is likely to increase in the coming decades as we live longer. The lifetime risk of developing atrial fibrillation and the related condition atrial flutter is about 25 percent in those who reach the age of forty. See Donald M. Lloyd-Jones et al., "Lifetime risk for development of atrial fibrillation: The Framingham Heart Study," *Circulation* 110 (2004), pp. 1042–1046; Gerald V. Naccarelli et al., "Increasing prevalence of atrial fibrillation and flutter in the United States," *American Journal of Cardiology* 104 (2009), pp. 1534–1539; Jan Heeringa et al., "Prevalence, incidence and lifetime risk of atrial fibrillation:

The Rotterdam study," *European Heart Journal* (*Eur Heart J*) 27 (2006), pp. 949–953.

2 It is estimated that about one in every five strokes is due to atrial fibrillation. See Paulus Kirchhof et al., "Outcome parameters for trials in atrial fibrillation, executive summary: Recommendation from a consensus conference organized by the German Atrial Fibrillation Competence NETwork (AFNET) and the European Heart Rhythm Association (EHRA)," *Eur Heart J* 28 (2007), pp. 2803–2817; Alan S. Go et al., "Prevalence of diagnosed atrial fibrillation in adults: National implications for rhythm management and stroke prevention: The Anticoagulation and Risk Factors in Atrial Fibrillation (ATRIA) Study," *Journal of the American Medical Association* (*JAMA*) 285 (2001), pp. 2370–2375; Stefan Knecht et al., "Atrial fibrillation in stroke-free patients is associated with memory impairment and hippocampal atrophy," *Eur Heart J* 29 (2008), pp. 2125–2132. Treatment includes anticoagulation that helps prevent the development of clots in the heart; see Elaine M. Hylek et al., "Effect of intensity of oral anticoagulation on stroke severity and mortality in atrial fibrillation," *New England Journal of Medicine* (*NEJM*) 349 (2003), pp. 1019–1026; Robert G. Hart, Lesly A. Pearce, Maria I. Aguilar, "Meta-analysis: Antithrombotic therapy to prevent stroke in patients who have nonvalvular atrial fibrillation," *Annals of Internal Medicine* (*Ann Intern Med*) 146 (2007), pp. 857–867. New anticoagulants were approved in 2010 for treatment of atrial fibrillation that are easier to monitor and pose a somewhat lower risk of bleeding: Stuart J. Connolly et al., "Dabigatran versus warfarin in patients with atrial fibrillation," *NEJM* 361 (2009), pp. 1139–1151; Brian F. Gage, "Can we rely on RE-LY?" *NEJM* 361 (2009), pp. 1200–1202.

3 The relationship between high blood cholesterol and cardiovascular disease was first recognized in large epidemiological studies like the famous one conducted in Framingham, Massachusetts. In that study, local residents were followed for decades by researchers who assessed not only blood lipids like cholesterol, but also hypertension, diabetes, and personal habits, like smoking: Daniel Levy, Susan Brink, *A Change of Heart: How the People of Framingham, Massachusetts, Helped Unravel the Mysteries of Cardiovascular Disease* (New York: Alfred A. Knopf, 2005); Daniel Levy, "50 years of discovery: Medical milestones from the National Heart, Lung, and Blood Institute's Framingham Heart Study," Hackensack, NJ: Center for Bio-Medical Communication, 1999.

3   An excellent clinical overview on preventing a future heart attack with statin medications: Michael J. Domanski, "Primary prevention of coronary artery disease," *NEJM* 357 (2007), pp. 1543–1545.

4   Michelle Byrd had an unusual side effect of abdominal pain with the second medication for her blood pressure, described in Troy D. Schmidt and Kevin M. McGrath, "Angiotension-converting enzyme inhibitor angioedema of the intestine: A case report and review of the literature," *American Journal of the Medical Sciences* 324 (2002), pp. 106–108; Thomas J. Byrne et al., "Isolated visceral angioedema: An underdiagnosed complication of ACE inhibitors," *Mayo Clinic Proceedings* 75 (2000), pp. 1201–1204.

4   An analysis of therapy for high blood pressure showing a beneficial trend with intensive treatment as requested by Michelle Byrd. These data are not statistically significant but taken by some experts to favor tight control of blood pressure: Blood Pressure Lowering Treatment Trialists' Collaboration, "Effects of different regimens to lower blood pressure on major cardiovascular events in older and younger adults: Meta-analysis of randomised trials," *British Medical Journal* 336 (2008), doi:10.1136/bmj.39548.738368.BE.

5   Alex Miller's comments about "changing the goalposts" reflect evolving definitions of what is normal and abnormal blood pressure, and the cutoffs for treatment, by expert committees in the United States: Avram V. Chobanian et al., "The Seventh Report of the Joint National Committee on Prevention, Detection, Evaluation, and Treatment of High Blood Pressure: The JNC 7 Report," *JAMA* 289 (2003), pp. 2560–2572. It is noteworthy that there are different "goalposts" in Europe, more akin to the prior cutoffs in the United States: Giuseppe Mancia et al., "2007 Guidelines for the Management of Arterial Hypertension: The Task Force for the Management of Arterial Hypertension of the European Society of Hypertension (ESH) and of the European Society of Cardiology (ESC)," *Journal of Hypertension* 25 (2007), pp. 1105–1187. An excellent study of differences in patient and physician views on benefit versus risk in treating hypertension: Finlay A. McAlister et al., "When should hypertension be treated? The different perspectives of Canadian family physicians and patients," *Canadian Medical Association Journal* (*CMAJ*) 163 (2000), pp. 403–408.

6   The fundamentals of health literacy in assessing clinical information are presented in an excellent primer: Steven Woloshin, Lisa M. Schwartz, H. Gilbert Welch, *Know Your Chances: Understanding Health Statistics* (Berkeley: University of California Press, 2008).

CHAPTER 1: WHERE AM I IN THE NUMBERS?

10 Data on statin prescriptions are found in Jennifer Couzin-Frankel, "U.S. panel favors wider use of preventive drug treatment," *Science* 327 (2010), pp. 130–131; BMJ Group, "High cholesterol: Statins for people with heart disease," *Best Health*, September 14, 2009; Erica S. Spatz, Maureen E. Canavan, Mayur M. Desai, "From here to Jupiter: Identifying new patients for statin therapy using data from the 1999–2004 National Health and Nutrition Examination Survey," *Circulation: Cardiovascular Quality & Outcomes* 2 (2009), pp. 41–48; David Mann et al., "Trends in statin use and low-density lipoprotein cholesterol levels among U.S. adults: Impact of the 2001 National Cholesterol Education Program Guidelines," *Annals of Pharmacotherapy* 42 (2008), pp. 1208–1215.

10 The discovery of statin drugs and their development as therapeutics by one of the Japanese scientists central to the work: Akira Endo, "The discovery and development of HMG-CoA reductase inhibitors," *Journal of Lipid Research* 33 (1992), pp. 1569–1582.

11 Data on the frequency of muscle pain and inflammation from statin medications: Tisha R. Joy, Robert A. Hegele, "Narrative review: Statin-related myopathy," *Ann Intern Med* 150 (2009), pp. 858–868; Julia Hippisley-Cos, Carol Coupland, "Unintended effects of statins in men and women in England and Wales: Population based cohort study using the QResearch database," *BMJ* 340 (2010) c2197, doi:10.1136/bmj.c2197.

11 One of the key studies relevant to treatment of people with elevated cholesterol and no prior history of heart disease, like Susan Powell, is Ian Ford et al., "Long-term follow-up of the West of Scotland Coronary Prevention Study," *NEJM* 357 (2007), pp. 1477–1486.

12 Data on how many patients decline to take prescribed medication or do not adhere to the regimen: Lars Osterberg, Terrence Blaschke, "Adherence to medication," *NEJM* 353 (2005), pp. 487–497; Joshua S. Benner et al., "Long-term persistence in use of statin therapy in elderly patients," *JAMA* 288 (2002), pp. 455–461; Mark Peyrot et al., "Correlates of insulin injection omission," *Diabetes Care* 33 (2010), pp. 240–245; Susan Mackie, "The value of DNKs," *NEJM* 362 (2010), p. 1561; Stephen Smith, "Take as directed," *Boston Globe*, May 10, 2010; Nancy Houston Miller, "Compliance with treatment regimens in chronic asymptomatic diseases," *American Journal of Medicine* 102 (1997), pp. 43–49; Joyce A. Cramer, "Compliance with

contraceptives and other treatments," *Obstetrics & Gynecology* 88 (1996), pp. 4S–12S. For women prescribed bisphosphonates, calcium, and vitamin D: Pierre D. Delmas et al., "Effect of monitoring bone turnover markers on persistence with risedronate treatment of postmenopausal osteoporosis," *Journal of Clinical Endocrinology & Metabolism* 92 (2007), pp. 1296–1304; Ethel S. Siris et al., "Adherence to bisphosphonate therapy, vitamin D and calcium supplements and fracture rates in osteoporotic women: Relationship to vertebral and nonvertebral fractures from 2 U.S. claims databases," *Mayo Clinic Proceedings* 81 (2006), pp. 1013–1022; Enkhe Badamgarav, Lorraine A. Fitzpatric, "A new look at osteoporosis outcomes: The influence of treatment, compliance, persistence, and adherence," *Mayo Clinic Proceedings* 81 (2006), pp. 1009–1012; National Community Pharmacists Association, "Enhancing prescription medicine adherence: A national action plan," National Council on Patient Information and Education, Rockville, MD, August 2007, p. 7; Katherine Hobson, "How can you help the medicine go down? Too many people don't take the drugs they're supposed to: Tackling that problem could save a lot of money and a lot of lives," *Wall Street Journal*, March 28, 2011.

13　The availability bias is elegantly described in Amos Tversky, Daniel Kahneman, "The framing of decisions and the psychology of choice," *Science* 211 (1981), pp. 453–458.

14　The bias in favor of natural approaches is found in Gretchen B. Chapman, "The psychology of medical decision making," in D. J. Koehler and N. Harvey (eds.), *Blackwell Handbook of Judgment and Decision Making* (Oxford, UK: Blackwell Publishing, 2004), pp. 585–603.

15　Loss aversion is described by Daniel Kahneman, Jack L. Knetsch, Richard H. Thaler, "The endowment effect, loss aversion, and status quo bias," *Journal of Economic Perspectives* 5 (1991), pp. 193–206. Also see Dan Ariely's lively discussion of loss aversion in *Predictably Irrational: The Hidden Forces That Shape Our Decisions* (New York: HarperCollins, 2008).

17　There are different risk calculators for heart attack; a reliable site that helped give Susan Powell understandable numbers: United States Department of Health and Human Services/National Heart, Lung, and Blood Institute, "Health Information for the Public," http://www.nhlbi.nih.gov/health.

18　The importance of calculating the "number needed to treat" is found in Steven Woloshin, Lisa M. Schwartz, H. Gilbert Welch, *Know Your Chances:*

Understanding Health Statistics (Berkeley: University of California Press, 2008). For more extensive commentary on the interpretation of number needed to treat, see Finlay A. McAlister et al., "Users' guides to the medical literature. Integrating research evidence with the care of the individual patient," *JAMA* 283 (2000), pp. 2829–2836; Finlay A. McAlister, "The 'number needed to treat' turns 20—and continues to be used and misused," *CMAJ* 179 (2008), pp. 549–553; Christopher A. K. Y. Chong et al., "An unadjusted NNT was a moderately good predictor of health benefit," *Journal of Clinical Epidemiology* 59 (2006), pp. 224–233; Peder Andreas Halvorsen, Ivar Sonbo Kristiansen, "Decisions on drug therapies by numbers needed to treat: A randomized trial," *Archives of Internal Medicine* 165 (2005), pp. 1140–1146; J. Nexoe, I. S. Kristiansen, D. Gyrd-Hansen, J. B. Nielsen, "Influence of number needed to treat, costs and outcome on preferences for a preventive drug," *Family Practice* 22 (2005), pp. 126–131; Arthur Marx, Heiner C. Bucher, "Numbers needed to treat derived from meta-analysis: A word of caution," *Evidence-Based Medicine* 8 (2003), pp. 36–37; Lonne Wen, Robert Badgett, John Cornell, "Number needed to treat: A descriptor for weighing therapeutic options," *American Journal of Health-System Pharmacy* 62 (2005), pp. 2031–2036.

18 Framing information and its impact on people's understanding of risk and their ultimate choice is found in Amos Tversky, Daniel Kahneman, "The framing of decisions and the psychology of choice," *Science* 211 (1981), pp. 453–458; Paul Slovic, "Perception of risk," *Science* 236 (1987), pp. 280–285. For the role of framing in medicine, see Barbara J. McNeil, Stephen G. Pauker, Harold C. Sox, Amos Tversky, "On the elicitation of preferences for alternative therapies," *NEJM* 306 (1982), pp. 1259–1269; Donald A. Redelmeier, Paul Rozin, Daniel Kahneman, "Understanding patients' decisions: Cognitive and emotional perspectives," *JAMA* 270 (1993), pp. 72–76.

20 The power of narratives by one of the cardinal researchers in learning and education: Howard Gardner, *Changing Minds: The Art and Science of Changing Our Own and Other People's Minds* (Boston: Harvard Business School Press, 2006).

20 How narratives versus data influence patient perceptions and choice: John B. F. de Wit, Enny Das, Raymond Vet, "What works best: Objective statistics or a personal testimonial? An assessment of the persuasive effects of different types of message evidence on risk perception," *Health Psychology* 27 (2008), pp. 110–115; Philip Broemer, "Ease of imagination moderates

reactions to differently framed health messages," *European Journal of Social Psychology* 34 (2004), pp. 103–119; Alexander J. Rothman, Peter Salovery, "Shaping perceptions to motivate healthy behavior: The role of message framing," *Psychological Bulletin* 121 (1997), pp. 3–19; Alexander J. Rothman, Nobert Schwarz, "Constructing perceptions of vulnerability: Personal relevance and the use of experiential information in health judgment," *Personality and Social Psychology Bulletin* 24 (1998), pp. 1053–1064; Michael D. Slater, Donna Rouner, "Value-affirmative and value-protective processing of alcohol education messages that include statistical evidence or anecdotes," *Communication Research* 23 (1996), pp. 210–235; Shelley E. Taylor, Suzanne C. Thomson, "Stalking the elusive 'vividness' effect," *Psychological Review* 89 (1982), pp. 155–181.

20 Much has been written about how drug advertising is designed and its impact on the public; see Steven Woloshin, Lisa M. Schwartz, Jennifer Tremmel, H. Gilbert Welch, "Direct-to-consumer advertisements for prescription drugs: What are Americans being sold?" *Lancet* 358 (2001), pp. 1141–1146; Dominick L. Frosch et al., "Creating demand for prescription drugs: A content analysis of television direct-to-consumer advertising," *Annals of Family Medicine* 5 (2007), pp. 6–13; Kurt C. Stange, "Doctor-patient and drug company–patient communication," *Annals of Family Medicine* 5 (2007), pp. 2–4; Kurt C. Stange, "Intended and unintended consequences of direct-to-consumer drug marketing," *Annals of Family Medicine* 5 (2007), pp. 175–178; Kate Pickert, "Do consumers understand drug ads?" *Time*, May 15, 2008; Ziad F. Gellad, Kenneth W. Lyles, "Direct-to-consumer advertising of pharmaceuticals," *American Journal of Medicine* 120 (2007), pp. 475–480; Julie M. Donohue, Marisa Cevasco, Meredith B. Rosenthal, "A decade of direct-to-consumer advertising of prescription drugs," *NEJM* 357 (2007), pp. 673–681; Ian D. Spatz, "Better drug ads, fewer side effects," *New York Times*, February 20, 2011. The lack of regulation of ads on the Internet is of particular concern: Bryan A. Liang, Timothy Mackey, "Direct-to-consumer advertising with interactive internet media: Global regulation and public health issues," *JAMA* 305 (2011), pp. 824–825. In addition, there is intense marketing of drugs to physicians; an excellent summary of its role in influencing how the doctor prescribes: Jeremy A. Greene, "Pharmaceutical marketing research and the prescribing physician," *Ann Intern Med* 146 (2007), pp. 742–748. An outstanding book on the pharmaceutical industry is Jerry Avorn, *Powerful Medicines: The Benefits, Risks, and Costs of Prescription Drugs* (New York: Alfred A. Knopf, 2004).

22 The study on exposure to television drug ads from the UCLA group: Dominick L. Frosch et al., "Creating demand for prescription drugs: A content analysis of television direct-to-consumer advertising," *Annals of Family Medicine* 5 (2007), pp. 6–13.

22 The references to the congressional committee is found in Kate Pickert, "Do consumers understand drug ads?" *Time*, May 15, 2008; Judy Foreman, "More specific drug ads, labels would help consumers, a study reveals," *Los Angeles Times*, June 8, 2009.

22 The study from the Dartmouth Institute for Health Policy and Clinical Practice: Lisa M. Schwartz et al., "Using a drug facts box to communicate drug benefits and harms: Two randomized trials," *Ann Intern Med* 150 (2009), pp. 516–527. Also see Jerry Avorn, "Communicating drug benefits and risks effectively: There must be a better way," *Ann Intern Med* 150 (2009), pp. 563–564; Jerry Avorn and Sebastian Schneeweiss, "Managing drug-risk information: What to do with all those new numbers," *NEJM* 361 (2009), pp. 647–649.

23 There is a rich literature on agreement and disagreement between patients and physicians about health priorities: Maida J. Sewitch et al., "Measuring differences between patients' and physicians' health perceptions: The patient-physician discordance scale," *Journal of Behavioral Medicine* 26 (2003), pp. 245–264; Eberhard Scheuer, Johann Steurer, Claus Buddeberg, "Predictors of differences in symptom perception of older patients and their doctors," *Family Practice* 19 (2002), pp. 357–361; Robert A. Bell et al., "Unmet expectations for care and the patient-physician relationship," *Journal of General Internal Medicine* (*JGIM*) 17 (2002), pp. 817–824; Joseph Greer, Richard Halgin, "Predictors of physician-patient agreement on symptoms etiology in primary care," *Psychosomatic Medicine* 68 (2006), pp. 277–282; Finlay A. McAlister et al., "When should hypertension be treated? The different perspectives of Canadian family physicians and patients," *CMAJ* 163 (2000), pp. 403–408; Roni Caryn Rabin, "Perceptions: Doctors, patients and a clash of priorities," *New York Times*, February 9, 2010.

25 Ronald M. Epstein, an eminent physician who advocates mindfulness in patient care, and Ellen Peters, a leading researcher in decision analysis, set forth the complexities of eliciting patient preferences in "Beyond information: Exploring patients' preferences," *JAMA* 302 (2009) pp. 195–197. See also Hilary A. Llewellyn-Thomas et al., "Studying patients' preferences in

health care decision making," *CMAJ* 147 (1992), pp. 859–864; Nick Sevdalis, Nigel Harvey, "Predicting preferences: A neglected aspect of shared decision-making," *Health Expectations* 9 (2006), pp. 245–251; Gretchen B. Chapman, "The psychology of medical decision making," in D. J. Koehler and N. Harvey (eds.), *Blackwell Handbook of Judgment and Decision Making* (Oxford, UK: Blackwell Publishing, 2004), pp. 585–603.

27   Each patient's personal preferences, needs, and values should be paramount in guiding care; see Institute of Medicine (National Academy of Sciences), *Crossing the Quality Chasm: A New Health System for the 21st Century* (Washington, DC: National Academy Press, 2001), http://www.nap.edu/books/0309072808/html. Also see Robert A. McNutt, "Shared medical decision making: Problems, process, progress," *JAMA* 292 (2002), pp. 2516–2518; Carla C. Keirns, Susan Dorr Goold, "Patient-centered care and preference-sensitive decision making," *JAMA* 302 (2009), pp. 1085–1086. This centrality of patient preference in choice, even when it conflicts with what a physician advises, is passionately presented by Dr. Donald Berwick (Donald Berwick, "What 'patient-centered' should mean: Confessions of an extremist," *Health Affairs—Web Exclusive* 28, no. 4 [2009], pp. W555–W565). See also Pamela Hartzband, Jerome Groopman, "Keeping the patient in the equation: Humanism and health care reform," *NEJM* 361 (2009), pp. 554–555.

27   Patient autonomy is a major subject of study. Its role in our culture is lucidly explored in Carl Schneider, *The Practice of Autonomy: Patients, Doctors, and Medical Decisions* (New York: Oxford University Press, 1998). See also Richard L. Street et al., "Patient participation in medical consultations: Why some patients are more involved than others," *Medical Care* 43 (2005), pp. 960–969.

Chapter 2: Believers and Doubters

[Jerry's Narrative]

32   Cholesterol as a risk factor in developing atherosclerosis was a prominent and controversial topic in the media: Leonard Engel, "Cholesterol: Guilty or innocent?" *New York Times*, May 12, 1963.

32   The history of elevated cholesterol as well as smoking predisposing to heart disease: Daniel Levy, Susan Brink, *A Change of Heart: How the People of*

Framingham, Massachusetts, Helped Unravel the Mysteries of Cardiovascular Disease (New York: Alfred A. Knopf, 2005); Daniel Levy, *50 years of discovery: Medical milestones from the National Heart, Lung, and Blood Institute's Framingham Heart Study* (Hackensack, NJ: Center for Bio-Medical Communication, January 1999).

32 The report of the surgeon general: "The 1964 Report on Smoking and Health," http://profiles.nlm.nih.gov/ps/retrieve/Narrative/NN/p-nid/60.

36 The difficult road to developing bone marrow transplantation is beautifully articulated in the Nobel address of Dr. E. Donnall Thomas: E. Donnall Thomas, Autobiography, Nobelprize.org, http://nobelprize.org/nobel_ prizes/medicine/laureates/1990/thomas-autobio.html. The considerable advances that had been made in sustaining patients through this intensive treatment can be found in Ted A. Gooley et al., "Reduced mortality after allogeneic hematopoietic-cell transplantation," *NEJM* 363 (2010), pp. 2091–2101; John H. Kersey, "The role of allogeneic-cell transplantation in leukemia," *NEJM* 363 (2010), pp. 2158–2159.

37 Stephen Gould's essay can be accessed: Stephen Jay Gould, "The Median Isn't the Message," CancerGuide, http://cancerguide.org/median_not_ msg.html.

37 Dr. Lawrence Einhorn pioneered the use of cisplatinum in the treatment of testicular cancer. His work is included in the story of Lance Armstrong's treatment in his book *It's Not About the Bike: My Journey Back to Life*, Rei Rep, ed. (New York: Berkley Trade, 2001).

39 The story of my back surgery and rehabilitation is told in *The Anatomy of Hope* (New York: Random House, 2005). An overview of conservative and aggressive measures for chronic back pain is found in Jerome Groopman, "A knife in the back: Is surgery the best approach to chronic back pain?" *New Yorker*, April 8, 2002.

[Pam's Narrative]

41 Dr. F. Truby King wrote influential books, now out of print: *Feeding and Care of Baby*, 1913; *The Expectant Mother and Baby's First Month: For Parents and Nurses*, 1923.

44 The findings of the Framingham study on estrogen: Peter W. F. Wilson, Robert J. Garrison, William P. Castelli, "Postmenopausal estrogen use, cigarette smoking, and cardiovascular morbidity in women over 50," *NEJM*

313 (1985), pp. 1038–1043. Also see: Stephen Hulley et al., "Randomized trial of estrogen plus progestin for secondary prevention of coronary heart disease in postmenopausal women," *JAMA* 280 (1998), pp. 605–613; Heart and Estrogen/Progestin Replacement Study Follow-up (HERS II), "Cardiovascular disease outcomes during 6.8 years of hormone therapy," *JAMA* 288 (2002), pp. 49–57.

44 The controversy about hormone replacement therapy for women at the time of menopause and after menopause continues: Andrea Z. LaCroix et al., "Health outcomes after stopping conjugated equine estrogens among post-menopausal women with prior hysterectomy: A randomized controlled trial," *JAMA* 305 (2011), pp. 1305–1314; Emily S. Jungheim, Graham A. Colditz, "Short-term use of unopposed estrogen: A balance of inferred risks and benefits," *JAMA* 305 (2011), pp. 1354–1355. The media follows the debate closely. Two excellent articles that represent the range of expert views: Gail Collins, "Medicine on the move," *New York Times* (op-ed), April 7, 2011; Tara Parker-Pope, "Estrogen lowers breast cancer and heart attack risk in some," *New York Times* (Well), April 6, 2011.

45 The diagnosis and treatment of Graves' disease is detailed in chapter 3. An excellent recent review is Gregory A. Brent, "Graves' disease," *NEJM* 358 (2008), pp. 2594–2605.

46 Pam's mother's advice about eating blueberries is featured in Frank Bruni's article about other octogenarians: Frank Bruni, "Death takes a rain check: How many blueberries a day does it take to keep the grim reaper away? An 87-year-old billionaire's quest to live forever—or at least to 125," *New York Times Magazine*, March 6, 2011.

CHAPTER 3: BUT IS IT BEST FOR ME?

51 There are nuances to the treatment of Graves' disease that need to be weighed in certain cases, like the size of the thyroid gland and whether there are associated eye abnormalities (called Graves' ophthalmopathy). An excellent overview of hyperthyroidism due to Graves' disease is Gregory A. Brent, "Graves' disease," *NEJM* 358 (2008), pp. 2594–2605.

52 Patrick Baptiste was treated for his diabetes by different specialists who had varying views on how to regulate his blood sugar. In this regard, it is notable that expert groups have differed on several aspects of the monitoring and treatment of diabetes, despite access to the same "evidence" from research

studies; see Jako S. Burgers et al., "Inside guidelines: Comparative analysis of recommendations and evidence in diabetes guidelines from 13 countries," *Diabetes Care* 25 (2002), pp. 1933–1939; Finlay A. McAlister et al., "How evidence-based are the recommendations in evidence-based guidelines?" *PLoS Medicine* 4 (2007), pp. 1325–1332.

52 The tight regulation of blood glucose with insulin and oral medications is an area of active research and differing opinions among specialists; see NICE-SUGAR Study Investigators, "Intensive versus conventional glucose control in critically ill patients," *NEJM* 360 (2009), pp. 1283–1297; Silvio E. Inzucchi, Mark D. Siegel, "Glucose control in the ICU: How tight is too tight?" *NEJM* 360 (2009), pp. 1346–1349; Action to Control Cardiovascular Risk in Diabetes Study Group, "Effects of intensive glucose lowering in Type 2 diabetes," *NEJM* 358 (2008), pp. 2545–2559; ADVANCE Collaborative Group, "Intensive blood glucose control and vascular outcomes in patients with Type 2 diabetes," *NEJM* 358 (2008), pp. 2560–2572; Robert G. Dluhy, Graham T. McMahon, "Intensive glycemic control in the ACCORD and ADVANCE trials," *NEJM* 358 (2008), pp. 2630–2633.

53 The randomized study of different therapies for Graves' disease: Ove Torring et al., "Graves' hyperthyroidism: Treatment with antithyroid drugs, surgery, or radioiodine—a prospective, randomized study: Thyroid Study Group," *Journal of Clinical Endocrinology & Metabolism* 81 (1996), pp. 2986–2993.

53 Differences between physician and patient preferences are addressed in Kate Cox et al., "Patients' involvement in decisions about medicines: GPs' perceptions of their preferences," *British Journal of General Practice* 57 (2007), pp. 777–784; Arthur S. Elstein, Gretchen B. Chapman, Sara J. Knight, "Patients' values and clinical substituted judgments: The case of localized prostate cancer," *Health Psychology* 24 (2005), pp. S85–S92; Susan M. Sawyer, H. John Fardy, "Bridging the gap between doctors' and patients' expectations of asthma management," *Journal of Asthma* 40 (2003), pp. 131–138; A. Spoorenberg et al., "Measuring disease activity in ankylosing spondylitis: Patient and physician have different perspectives," *Rheumatology* (Oxford) 44 (2005), pp. 789–795.

54 The geographic variation in approaches to treatment of Graves' disease: Leonard Wartofsky et al., "Differences and similarities in the diagnosis and treatment of Graves' disease in Europe, Japan, and the United States," *Thyroid* 1 (1991), pp. 129–135; Daniel Glinoer et al., "The management of hyper-

thyroidism due to Graves' disease in Europe in 1986: Results of an international survey," *Acta Endocrino Logica* 185 (Suppl.) (1987), pp. 9–37; Barbara Solomin et al., "Current trends in the management of Graves' disease," *Journal of Clinical Endocrinology & Metabolism* 70 (1990), pp. 1518–1524; Y. Nagayama, M. Izumi, S. Nagataki, "The management of hyperthyroidism due to Graves' disease in Japan in 1988: The Japan Thyroid Association," *Endocrinologica Japonica* 36 (1989), pp. 299–314.

54   Daniel Bernoulli's work in probability theory: W. W. Rouse Ball, *A Short Account of the History of Mathematics*, 4th ed. (Mineola, NY: Dover Publications, 2010); and http://www-history.mcs.st-and.ac.uk/Biographies/ Bernoulli_Daniel.html. The formula for expected utility: Alan Schwartz, George Bergus, *Medical Decision Making: A Physician's Guide* (Cambridge, UK: Cambridge University Press, 2008).

54   An examination of the methodology of determining utilities and preferences can be found in Alan Schwartz, George Bergus, *Medical Decision Making: A Physician's Guide* (Cambridge, UK: Cambridge University Press, 2008); George W. Torrance, "Measurement of health state utilities for economic appraisal: A review," *Journal of Health Economics* 5 (1986), pp. 1–30.

55   The complexity of trying to project future feelings has been studied extensively in cognitive psychology; see George Loewenstein, David Schkade, "Wouldn't it be nice? Predicting future feelings," in D. Kahneman, E. Diener, and N. Schwarz (eds.), *Well-Being: The Foundation of Hedonic Psychology* (New York: Russell Sage Foundation, 1998), pp. 85–105. Also see Norman F. Boyd et al., "Whose utilities for decision analysis?" *Medical Decision Making* 10 (1990), pp. 58–67; Nick Sevdalis, Nigel Harvey, "Predicting preferences: A neglected aspect of shared decision-making," *Health Expectations* 9 (2006), pp. 245–251. The dilemma of forecasting is wonderfully illuminated in Daniel Gilbert, *Stumbling on Happiness* (New York: Vintage Books, 2007).

57   Constructing preferences "on the spot" is addressed in Sarah Lichtenstein and Paul Slovic, "The Construction of Preference: An Overview," in Lichtenstein and Slovic (eds.), *The Construction of Preference* (New York: Cambridge University Press, 2006). See also Ronald M. Epstein, Ellen Peters, "Beyond information: Exploring patients' preferences," *JAMA* 302 (2009), pp. 195–197.

57   The importance of the default option and how it may be used in changing health behaviors and other social issues: Richard H. Thaler, Cass R. Sun-

stein, *Nudge: Improving Decisions About Health, Wealth, and Happiness* (New York, Penguin Books, 2009).

58 On the challenge of teaching physicians and other health care professionals how to elicit preferences in an objective manner while providing clear information, see Ronald M. Epstein, Ellen Peters, "Beyond information: Exploring patients' preferences," *JAMA* 302 (2009), pp. 195–197. For differences in how patients and physicians weigh the importance of facts about clinical problems and the goals and concerns about available treatments: Karen R. Sepucha et al., "Developing instruments to measure the quality of decisions: Early results for a set of symptom-driven decisions," *Patient Education and Counseling* 73 (2008), pp. 504–510; Karen Sepucha et al., "An approach to measuring the quality of breast cancer decisions," *Patient Education and Counseling* 65 (2007), pp. 261–269.

59 The studies cited on atrial fibrillation are P. J. Devereaux et al., "Differences between perspectives of physicians and patients on anticoagulation in patients with atrial fibrillation: Observational study," *BMJ* 323 (2001), pp. 1218–1222; Malcolm Man-Son-Hing et al., "The effect of qualitative vs. quantitative presentation of probability estimates on patient decision-making: A randomized trial," *Health Expectations* 5 (2002), pp. 246–255.

60 The new anticoagulant approved by the FDA in 2010: Stuart J. Connolly et al., "Dabigatran versus warfarin in patients with atrial fibrillation," *NEJM* 361 (2009), pp. 1139–1151; Brian F. Gage, "Can we rely on RE-LY?" *NEJM* 361 (2009), pp. 1200–1202. Also see Stuart J. Connolly et al., "Apixaban in patients with atrial fibrillation," *NEJM* (Online First, February 10, 2011). The risks and benefits of bleeding versus stroke prevention: B. Nhi Beasley, Ellis F. Unger, Robert Temple, "Anticoagulant options: Why the FDA approved a higher but not a lower dose of dabigatran," *NEJM* (Online First, April 13, 2011).

The application of Bernoulli's formula to atrial fibrillation is even more complicated because accurate information about the first part of the formula, the probability of an outcome, is not available for an individual; it is available only for groups of patients. For example, age, gender, genetics, lifestyle, diet, concurrent medical conditions, and a host of other variables all influence the probability of stroke or hemorrhage while on anticoagulation treatment. Dr. Liana Fraenkel and Dr. Terri Fried of the Yale School of Medicine wrote an insightful article on how hard it is to give individual patients with atrial fibrillation accurate information on their risk of bleeding from anticoagulation treatment. This is particularly true for the elderly or those who have coexisting common medical problems, like diabetes, kidney disease, and difficulty with balance, because the data on risks and benefits of anticoagulation come from studies that typically exclude these kinds of patients: Liana Fraenkel, Terri R. Fried, "Individualized medical decision making," *Archives of Internal Medicine* 170 (2010), pp. 566–569.

61 Number needed to harm is discussed in Finlay A. McAlister et al., "Users' guides to the medical literature. Integrating research evidence with the care of the individual patient," *JAMA* 283 (2000), pp. 2829–2836; Finlay A. McAlister, "The 'number needed to treat' turns 20—and continues to be used and misused," *CMAJ* 179 (2008), pp. 549–553.

61 The study on physician and patient assessment of when to be treated for high blood pressure: Finlay A. McAlister et al., "When should hypertension be treated? The different perspectives of Canadian family physicians and patients," *CMAJ* 163 (2000), pp. 403–408.

62 Hypertension guidelines and cutoffs are found in Avram V. Chobanian et al., "The Seventh Report of the Joint National Committee on Prevention, Detection, Evaluation, and Treatment of High Blood Pressure: The JNC 7 Report," *JAMA* 289 (2003), pp. 2560–2572; Giuseppe Mancia et al., "2007 Guidelines for the Management of Arterial Hypertension: The Task Force for the Management of Arterial Hypertension of the European Society of Hypertension (ESH) and of the European Society of Cardiology (ESC)," *Journal of Hypertension* 25 (2007), pp. 1105–1187. See also Hector O. Ventura, Carl J. Lavie, "Antihypertensive therapy for prehypertension: Relationship with cardiovascular outcomes," *JAMA* 305 (2011), pp. 940–941. Numbers relevant to Alex Miller's case: One first should distinguish between the absolute benefit versus relative reduction with treatment. Mild hypertension with a diastolic reading of 90 to 100, based on seventeen controlled trials, with most people younger than sixty-five years old, showed a 16 percent relative reduction in coronary events and a 40 percent relative reduction in stroke. But the absolute benefit is related to the predicted number of cardiovascular complications. You need to treat four to five years to prevent a coronary event in 0.7 percent of patients and prevent a stroke in 1.3 percent of patients, for a total of 2 percent, with a decrease in mortality of 0.8 percent. So to calculate the number needed to treat, you need to treat one hundred patients with antihypertensive medication for four to five years to prevent cardiovascular complications in two of them. Flipping the frame,

this means that ninety-eight people do not benefit from the therapy out of one hundred treated. Systolic hypertension is most relevant to the elderly, where it's often an isolated finding without elevation in the diastolic reading. Here, you need to treat eighteen older patients for five years to prevent a cardiovascular complication in one, meaning that seventeen of eighteen people who are elderly treated with medication do not clearly benefit. An excellent overview of patients' understanding these data and making choices for therapy of hypertension: H. Gilbert Welch, *Overdiagnosed: Making People Sick in the Pursuit of Health* (Boston: Beacon Press, 2011). It is noteworthy that Europeans have a different definition of what hypertension is, with cutoffs that are 5 to 10 millimeters of mercury higher than those in the United States. This is in part because of how different experts who guide committees view the same database with regard to defining a malady and, importantly, how they weigh the risks and benefits of treatment.

62 Rodney Hayward's important article is in Kerianne H. Quanstrum, Rodney A. Hayward, "Lessons from the mammography wars," *NEJM* 363 (2010), pp. 1076–1079. Also see Finlay A. McAlister, "Applying evidence to patient care: From black and white to shades of grey," *Ann Intern Med* 138 (2003), pp. 938–939; Carla C. Keirns, Susan Dorr Goold, "Patient-centered care and preference-sensitive decision making," *JAMA* 302 (2009), pp. 1085–1086.

63 In addition, "arbitrary" cutoffs for treatment of atrial fibrillation are discussed in Liana Fraenkel, Terri R. Fried, "Individualized medical decision making," *Archives of Internal Medicine* 170 (2010), pp. 566–569.

63 For a discussion of guidelines and their limitations, see Allan D. Sniderman, Curt D. Furberg, "Why guideline-making requires reform," *JAMA* 301 (2009), pp. 429–431; John P. A. Ioannidis, "Contradicted and initially stronger effects in highly cited clinical research," *JAMA* 294 (2005), pp. 218–228; Mary E. Tinetti, "Potential pitfalls of disease-specific guidelines for patients with multiple conditions," *NEJM* 351 (2004), pp. 2870–2874; Patrick J. O'Connor, "Adding value to evidence-based clinical guidelines," *JAMA* 294 (2005), pp. 741–743; Finlay A. McAlister et al., "Users' guides to the medical literature. Integrating research evidence with the care of the individual patient," *JAMA* 283 (2000), pp. 2829–2836; Patrick Conway, Carolyn Clancy, "Comparative-effectiveness research: Implications of the federal coordinating council's report," *NEJM* 361 (2009), pp. 328–330; Jerome Groopman, *How Doctors Think* (New York: Houghton Mifflin, 2007); Pamela Hartzband, Jerome Groopman, "Keeping the patient in the

equation: Humanism and health care reform," *NEJM* 361 (2009), pp. 554–555; Jerome Groopman, "Health care: Who knows 'best'?" *New York Review of Books* 57 (2010), pp. 12–15; Editorial, "Guiding the guidelines," *Lancet* 377 (2011), p. 1125. Because of the many limitations of guidelines, some researchers propose "individualized" guidelines. These are centered on outcome and cost but do not include detailed utility assessment: David M. Eddy et al., "Individualized guidelines: The potential for increasing quality and reducing costs," *Ann Intern Med* 154 (2011), pp. 627–634.

64 There are differing expert recommendations about how to treat elevated cholesterol levels in adults, including "Third Report of the National Cholesterol Education Program (NCEP) Expert Panel on Detection, Evaluation, and Treatment of High Blood Cholesterol in Adults (Adult Treatment Panel III)," *Circulation* 106 (2002), pp. 3143–3421; Uli C. Broedl, Hans-Christian Geiss, Klaus G. Parhofer, "Comparison of current guidelines for primary prevention of coronary heart disease," *JGIM* 18 (2003), pp. 190–195. This study done in Germany of one hundred consecutive people seen in a clinic for elevated cholesterol analyzed whether each patient would be treated with a statin drug according to one set of guidelines in the United States versus a set of guidelines shared among European countries and a third set developed in the United Kingdom. Twice as many Americans would have a statin drug recommended to treat their elevated cholesterol compared with Europeans and more than twice as many compared with people in England, Scotland, and Wales. This is not because American physicians who formulate these recommendations are smarter or more ignorant than their counterparts or that one expert group is working from a different database compared with another group. All three of the expert committees were analyzing the information primarily from large multiyear clinical studies. Rather, differences in recommendations reflect differences in weighing the value of the treatment in preventing certain cardiovascular problems versus the risks of the medications and, to be sure, their costs.

64 Potential conflicts of interest among experts who craft guidelines: Institute of Medicine. *Conflict of Interest in Medical Research, Education, and Practice* (Washington, DC: National Academies Press, 2009); Pamela Hartzband, Jerome Groopman, "Keeping the patient in the equation: Humanism and health care reform, *NEJM* 361 (2009), pp. 554–555; Courtney Humphries, "Deeply conflicted: How can we insulate ourselves from conflicts of interest? The most popular solution—disclosing them—turns out not to help," *Boston Globe,* May 15, 2011.

64 Ongoing controversy around such guidelines and the risks-versus-benefits effects of statins are found in Jennifer Couzin, "Cholesterol veers off script," *Science* 322 (2008), pp. 220–223; J. Abramson, J. M. Wright, "Are lipid-lowering guidelines evidence-based?" *Lancet* 369 (2007), pp. 168–169; Nortin M. Hadler, *Worried Sick: A Prescription for Health in an Overtreated America* (Chapel Hill: University of North Carolina Press, 2008). The issue of treating to maximally lower the LDL levels: Study of the Effectiveness of Additional Reductions in Cholesterol and Homocysteine (SEARCH) Collaborative Group, "Intensive lowering of LDL cholesterol with 80 mg versus 20 mg simvastatin daily in 12064 survivors of myocardial infarction: A double-blind randomised trial," *Lancet* 376 (2010), pp. 1658–1669; Bernard M. Y. Cheung, Karen S. L. Lam, "Is intensive LDL-cholesterol lowering beneficial and safe?" *Lancet* 376 (2010), pp. 1622–1623; Rodney A. Hayward, Timothy P. Hofer, Sandeep Vijan, "Narrative review: Lack of evidence for recommended low-density lipoprotein treatment targets: A solvable problem," *Ann Intern Med* 145 (2006), pp. 520–530.

64 The durability of one hundred recommendations from expert committees: Kaveh G. Shojania et al., "How quickly do systematic reviews go out of date? A survival analysis," *Ann Intern Med* 147 (2007), pp. 224–233. Also see Paul G. Shekelle et al., "Validity of the Agency for Healthcare Research and Quality clinical practice guidelines: How quickly do guidelines become outdated?" *JAMA* 286 (2001), pp. 1461–1467. Suspending practice guidelines at five years: Amir Qaseem et al., "The development of clinical practice guidelines and guidance statements of the American College of Physicians: Summary of methods," *Ann Intern Med* 153 (2010), pp. 194–199.

65 The controversy about hormonal replacement therapy for postmenopausal women continues; see Rowan T. Chlebowski et al., "Estrogen plus progestin and breast cancer incidence and mortality in postmenopausal women," *JAMA* 304 (2010), pp. 1684–1692; Peter B. Bach, "Postmenopausal hormone therapy and breast cancer: An uncertain trade-off," *JAMA* 304 (2010), pp. 1719–1720. Also see recent debate over estrogen replacement for women who had a hysterectomy: Andrea Z. LaCroix et al., "Health outcomes after stopping conjugated equine estrogens among postmenopausal women with prior hysterectomy: A randomized controlled trial," *JAMA* 305 (2011), pp. 1305–1314; Emily S. Jungheim, Graham A. Colditz, "Short-term use of unopposed estrogen: A balance of inferred risks and benefits," *JAMA* 305 (2011), pp. 1354–1355.

Regarding women's health, there also is debate among experts about the indications for bisphosphonate medications: Murray J. Favus, "Bisphosphonates for osteoporosis," *NEJM* 363 (2010), pp. 2027–2035; Natasha Singer, "Questions for doctors, and juries: Cases cast doubt on frequent use of bone-loss drugs," *New York Times*, November 11, 2010.

65   Another example of the complexity of applying guidelines involves asthma treatment and real world practice: David Price et al., "Leukotriene antagonists as first-line or add-on asthma-controller therapy," *NEJM* 364 (2011), pp. 1695–1707; Sven-Erik Dahlen, Barbro Dahlen, Jeffrey M. Drazen, "Asthma treatment guidelines meet the real world," *NEJM* (editorial) 364 (2011), pp. 1769–1770; James H. Ware, Mary Beth Harmel, "Pragmatic trials—Guides to better patient care?" *NEJM* 364 (2011), pp. 1685–1687.

65   Informed patient preferences at the "pinnacle" of quality care: Institute of Medicine (National Academy of Sciences), *Crossing the Quality Chasm: A New Health System for the 21st Century* (Washington, DC: National Academy Press, 2001), http://www.nap.edu/books/0309072808/html.

65   Between November 2006 and May 2007, researchers at the University of Michigan conducted a national survey of medical decisions, contacting by telephone at random 3,100 adults forty years and older in the United States. Participants were asked a series of questions about nine common medical decisions they might have discussed with their doctors in the previous two years. These medical decisions included initiating prescription medications for high blood pressure, elevated cholesterol, or depression; screening tests for colorectal, breast, or prostate cancer; and surgeries for low back pain, cataracts, or knee or hip replacement. Of these nine decisions, 82 percent of the people surveyed had made at least one in the preceding two years, and 56 percent had made two or more. Seventy-two percent had discussed at least one cancer screening test, 43 percent considered taking at least one of the medications, and 16 percent had discussed one or more of the surgical interventions. There were approximately 130 million adults aged forty years and older in the United States in July 2006, so extrapolating from the survey, about 33 million adults discussed initiating medication for elevated cholesterol, 27 million for high blood pressure, and 16 million for depression; more than 10 million considered cataract surgery and about 7 million considered an operation for low back pain or to replace a diseased knee or

hip. Less than half the patients recalled being asked about their preferences regarding cholesterol medications or blood pressure medications. This finding contrasted with patient reports that in more than 80 percent of instances, the physician expressed his opinion about initiating drug treatment for hypertension or elevated cholesterol. About a fifth of the patients did not recall being asked their preferences for surgery for low back pain or joint replacement. Perhaps most striking was that in the discussion between the doctor and patient, a disconnect occurred in presenting the pros and cons of therapy: in more than 90 percent of cases, there was a discussion of benefits of treatment (pros or "reasons to act") for medicating high blood pressure or elevated cholesterol, but in less than 50 percent the cons or "reasons not to act" were discussed. Discussions about surgery were more balanced, with 60 percent of the cons aired for hip or knee replacement, 80 percent for low back surgery, and about 40 percent for cataracts. Thus overall, discussions were weighted toward reasons to act much more frequently than reasons not to act. See: Brian J. Zikmund-Fisher et al, "The decision study: A nationwide survey of United States adults regarding 9 common medical decisions," *Medical Decision Making* 30 (2010), pp. S20–S34; Brian J. Zikmund-Fisher et al., "The decision study: A nationwide survey of United States adults regarding 9 common medical decisions," *Med Decis Making* 30 (2010), pp. S20–S34; Brian J. Zikmund-Fisher et al., "Deficits and variations in patients' experience with making 9 common medical decisions: The decisions survey," *Med Decis Making* 30 (2010), pp. S85–S95; Neda Ratanawangsa et al., "Race, ethnicity, and shared decision making for hyperlipidemia and hypertension treatment: The decisions survey," *Med Decis Making* 30 (2010), pp. S65–S76. A critique of the survey: Stephen G. Pauker, "Medical decision making: How patients choose," *Med Decis Making* 30 (2010), pp. S8–S10. An analysis of its implications: Floyd J. Fowler, Jr., Carrie A. Levin, Karen R. Sepucha, "Informing and involving patients to improve the quality of medical decisions," *Health Affairs* 30 (2011), pp. 699–707.

66 There is a powerful imperative to standardize medical care and follow guidelines strictly; see Stephen J. Swensen et al., "Cottage industry to postindustrial care: The revolution in health care delivery," *NEJM* 362 (2010), pp. E12(1)–E12(4); Robert H. Brook, "A physician = emotion + passion + science," *JAMA* 304 (2010), pp. 2528–2529; David Leonhardt, "Making health care better," *New York Times Magazine*, November 8, 2009. For a humanistic view of care, see Abraham Verghese, "Treat the patient, not the CT

scan," *New York Times*, February 27, 2011; Pamela Hartzband, Jerome Groopman, "Keeping the patient in the equation: Humanism and health care reform," *NEJM* 361 (2009), pp. 554–555.

66   The importance of standardization in safety measures and emergency care: Susan Dentzer, "Still crossing the quality chasm—or suspended over it?" *Health Affairs* 30 (2011), pp. 554–555; Debabrata Mukherjee, "Implementation of evidence-based therapies for myocardial infarction and survival," *JAMA* (editorial) 305 (2011), pp. 1710–1711. A poignant recounting of the origins of the patient safety movement, told in a mother's voice: Sorrel King, *Josie's Story: A Mother's Inspiring Crusade to Make Medical Care Safe* (New York, NY: Atlantic Monthly Press, 2009).

CHAPTER 4: REGRET

70   An overview of systemic lupus erythematosus, an autoimmune disease, and patients who achieve long-term remission like Lisa Norton: Josef S. Smolen, "Therapy of systemic lupus erythematosus: A look into the future," *Arthritis Research* 4 (Suppl. 3) (2002), pp. S25–S30; Murray B. Urowitz et al., "Prolonged remission in systemic lupus erythematosus," *Journal of Rheumatology* 32 (2005), pp. 1467–1472.

71   A history of natural healing is found in the excellent book by Anne Harrington, *The Cure Within: A History of Mind-Body Medicine* (New York: W. W. Norton & Co., 2008). See also Andrew Weil, *Spontaneous Healing: How to Discover and Enhance Your Body's Natural Ability to Maintain and Heal Itself* (New York: Alfred A. Knopf, 1995). The comment by Lisa Norton about her "wacky books" calls to mind a famous and contested case of remission of autoimmune disease following bed rest and humor; see Norman Cousins, *Anatomy of an Illness as Perceived by the Patient* (New York: Bantam Doubleday Dell, 1981). Dr. Howard Spiro, a gastroenterologist at the Yale School of Medicine, analyzed Cousins's story and speculated it might be a misdiagnosis in *The Power of Hope: A Doctor's Perspective* (New Haven, CT: Yale University Press, 1998).

75   The importance of recognizing making decisions when "hot" and when "cold" is found in George Loewenstein, "Hot-cold empathy gaps and medical decision making," *Health Psychology* 24 (2005), pp. S49–S56; also see Paul Slovic et al., "Affect, risk, and decision making," *Health Psychology* 24 (2005), pp. S35–S40; Sarah Lichtenstein and Paul Slovic, "The Construc-

tion of Preference: An Overview," in Lichtenstein and Slovic (eds.), *The Construction of Preference* (New York: Cambridge University Press, 2006).

75   There has been considerable research over the past decade trying to distinguish between beneficial effects of surgery versus placebo in alleviating pain and improving function in the treatment of arthritic joints, particularly the knee; see David T. Felson, Joseph Buckwalter, "Debridement and lavage for osteoarthritis of the knee," *NEJM* 347 (2002), pp. 132–133; Brian R. Wolf, Joseph A. Buckwalter, "Randomized surgical trials and 'sham' surgery: Relevance to modern orthopaedics and minimally invasive surgery," *Iowa Orthopaedic Journal* 26 (2006), pp. 107–111; J. Bruce Moseley et al., "A controlled trial of arthroscopic surgery for osteoarthritis of the knee," *NEJM* 347 (2002), pp. 81–88. The variable course of bone-on-bone arthritis of the knee is highlighted in the vignette by Dr. Donald Berwick in "My right knee," *Ann Intern Med* 142 (2005), pp. 121–125. Also see Thomas M. Burton, "New doubts about popular joint surgery," *Wall Street Journal*, October 14, 2008.

77   There is extensive literature on regret and decision making. For work by Daniel Kahneman and Amos Tversky related to investment and regret, see Daniel Kahneman, Amos Tversky, "The psychology of preferences," *Scientific American* 246 (1982), pp. 160–173; Daniel Kahneman, Dale T. Miller, "Norm theory: Comparing reality to its alternatives," *Psychological Review* 93 (1986), pp. 136–153. The example of regret in team sports is from Marcel Zeelenberg et al., "The inaction effect in the psychology of regret," *Journal of Personality and Social Psychology* 82 (2002), pp. 314–327.

77   Several other excellent articles relevant to the experiences of Lisa Norton and Carl Simpson are Terry Connolly et al., "Regret and responsibility in the evaluation of decision outcomes," *Organizational Behavior and Human Decision Processes* 70 (1997), pp. 73–85; Terry Connolly, David Butler, "Regret in economic and psychological theories of choice," *Journal of Behavioral Decision Making* 19 (2006), pp. 139–154; Terry Connolly, Jochen Reb, "Regret in cancer-related decisions," *Health Psychology* 24 (2005), pp. S29–S34; Hannah Faye Chua et al., "Decision-related loss: Regret and disappointment," *NeuroImage* 47 (2009), pp. 2031–2040. Regret is often characterized as irrational and an impediment to sound choices. But some researchers contend that anticipated regret can be "rational" if it approximates the degree of regret that one experiences in the future. Similarly, experienced regret is "rational" if one can learn from it. Several germane articles include Terry Connolly, Marcel Zeelenberg, "Regret in decision making," *Current*

Directions in Psychological Science 11 (2002), pp. 212–216; Marcel Zeelenberg et al., "Emotional reactions to the outcomes of decisions: The role of counterfactual thought in the experience of regret and disappointment," *Organizational Behavior and Human Decision Processes* 75 (1998), pp. 117–141; Marcel Zeelenberg et al., "The experience of regret and disappointment," *Cognition and Emotion* 12 (1998), pp. 221–230.

78 Marco daCosta DiBonaventura of Memorial Sloan-Kettering Cancer Center and Gretchen Chapman of Rutgers University explore a number of issues related to being vaccinated for influenza: "Do decision biases predict bad decisions? Omission bias, naturalness bias, and influenza vaccination," *Medical Decision Making* 28 (2008), pp. 532–539. Chapman relates this to different forecasting scenarios where there is short-term cost versus long-term gain: Gretchen B. Chapman et al., "Value for the future and preventive health behavior," *Journal of Experimental Psychology: Applied* 7 (2001), pp. 235–250.

80 The literature on patient emotions and physician relationships, relevant to patient feelings of disappointing the doctor, the power imbalance, and difficulty in challenging an expert: Vikki A. Entwistle et al., "Supporting patient autonomy: The importance of clinician-patient relationships," *JGIM* (Online First, March 6, 2010); Debra Roter, Judith A. Hall, *Doctors Talking with Patients/Patients Talking with Doctors* (Westport, CT: Praeger Publishing, 2006); and Jerome Groopman, *How Doctors Think* (New York: Houghton Mifflin, 2007).

81 The reader may surmise that Pam's mother is a deep doubter with a naturalism bias, while Jerry's mother was a believer, profoundly respectful of the medical profession and its technology.

83 Carl E. Schneider highlights the cultural pressures that may cause physicians to refrain from giving direct advice for fear of violating patient autonomy: Carl E. Schneider, *The Practice of Autonomy: Patients, Doctors, and Medical Decisions* (New York: Oxford University Press, 1998).

85 Dr. James Weinstein, an orthopedic surgeon at Dartmouth-Hitchcock Medical Center, is a leading advocate of shared medical decision making in approaching orthopedic surgery, where data on outcomes are often limited and where indications can vary significantly from patient to patient; see James N. Weinstein, Kate Clay, Tamara S. Morgan, "Informed patient choice: Patient-centered valuing of surgical risks and benefits," *Health Af-*

fairs 26 (2007), pp. 726–730; Barry Schwartz, Jim Weinstein, "Partnership: Doctor and patient," *Spine* 30 (2005), pp. 269–271.

CHAPTER 5: NEIGHBORLY ADVICE

87 Prostate cancer is the most commonly diagnosed malignancy other than skin cancer in the United States. In 2010, about 212,000 men received the diagnosis. Over the course of a lifetime, the risk of an American man developing prostate cancer is 16 percent, but the risk of dying of prostate cancer is 2.9 percent. These data indicate that prostate cancer often grows so slowly that most men die of other causes before the tumor becomes a problem. At the same time, among men found to have prostate cancer, when it is confined to the prostate and treated, survival free of the cancer at five years is 100 percent, while for those in whom the cancer has spread at time of diagnosis, with distant metastasis, five-year survival is about 32 percent. Thus, tumors that have spread are generally not curable. Data on prostate cancer incidence: Ahmedin Jemal et al., "Cancer Statistics, 2009," *Cancer* 59 (2009), pp. 225–249; Matthew R. Smith, "Effective treatment for early-stage prostate cancer—possible, necessary, or both?" *NEJM* (editorial) 364 (2011), pp. 1770–1772.

88 There is considerable debate about the use of PSA testing to screen for prostate cancer, reviewed in Michael J. Barry, "Screening for prostate cancer: The controversy that refuses to die," *NEJM* 360 (2009), pp. 1351–1354. The difficulty is in distinguishing between finding those aggressive cancers that, with treatment, will save men's lives and finding cancers that might never cause harm but are nonetheless treated, resulting in side effects of incontinence and impotence. Even after two recent large, randomized controlled trials, one conducted in Europe, the other in the United States, the issue of PSA testing is not settled.

The first of these recent trials is the European Randomized Study of Screening for Prostate Cancer, or ERSPC. The ERSPC evaluated 182,160 men between the ages of fifty and seventy-four who were randomly assigned to regular PSA screening, on average once every four years, or a control group that was not offered regular screening. The study used different recruiting and randomization procedures across seven centers in Europe. Furthermore, PSA cutoffs at which to perform a biopsy were not uniform but ranged between 2.5 and 4, with most centers using a cutoff at 3. There was incomplete information on how often the men in the control group at all centers had PSA screening done, although at one site in Rotterdam, the Netherlands, about a quarter of men in the control group had PSA testing. After nine years of follow-up, among men between the ages of fifty-five and sixty-nine, death from prostate cancer was 20 percent lower in the group that had regular screening. But again, we need to harken back to Susan Powell and look beyond the relative risk reduction of 20 percent to the "number needed to treat," or here, the number needed to be screened. This turned out to be 1,410 men needed to be screened to prevent 1 prostate cancer death over nine years. The number is so large because most men screened did not have prostate cancer. Of those who did have a cancer detected by PSA screening, 48 additional patients would need to be diagnosed with prostate cancer to prevent a single prostate cancer death—that is, despite the detection of cancer, there was a modest impact on saving lives (1 saved life, 48 lives not saved). The study did not address quality of life, so there was no information about the side effects of impotence or incontinence from radiation or surgery or from the psychological burden of knowing that you have a cancer and not treating it actively ("watchful waiting").

Critics of this European study pointed out that a substantial proportion of the control group received PSA testing, that about 25 percent of the cancers detected in the screening group did not receive curative treatment with either surgery or radiation, and since prostate cancer can grow very slowly, a follow-up of nine years to assess survival benefit may be too short; see Fritz H. Schroder et al., "Screening and prostate-cancer mortality in a randomized European study," *NEJM* 360 (2009), pp. 1320–1328.

The same issue of the *New England Journal of Medicine* carried the report from the Prostate, Lung, Colorectal, and Ovarian (PLCO) Cancer Screening Trial in the United States that found no benefit from annual PSA testing.

The PLCO study enrolled 76,693 men between the ages of fifty-five and seventy-four who were randomly assigned to annual screening with PSA and a digital rectal examination or to "usual care." The indications for biopsy were a PSA cutoff of 4 or an abnormal rectal examination. A very high proportion of the men in the "usual care" control group, more than 50 percent, underwent PSA testing. After seven years of follow-up, there was no reduction in death between the two groups. This negative result of the trial could be attributed to the high rate of PSA testing in the control group, the higher PSA cutoff of 4 compared with the European cutoff of 2.5 to 4, or the relatively short follow-up period; see Gerald L. Andriole et al., "Mortality results from a randomized prostate-cancer screening trial," *NEJM* 360 (2009), pp. 1310–1319.

There was considerable expectation in the medical community that these two large, randomized studies would yield results that would resolve the controversy about screening through PSA testing, but that proved not to be the case. It is unlikely the issue will be settled soon.

Another way to assess PSA testing is to ask how accurately it predicts prostate cancer in a man with no symptoms. This performance statistic is called the "positive predictive value," meaning the proportion of men with a PSA above the often used cutoff of 4 who will be found to have cancer. Overall, the positive predictive value for a PSA level greater than 4 is approximately 30 percent, meaning that a proportion slightly smaller than one in three men with this PSA level will have prostate cancer detected on biopsy. For PSA levels between 4 and 10, the positive predictive value is about the same, 25 percent. Only when PSA levels rise above 10 does the test better predict the presence of cancer, in 42 to 64 percent of men depending on the study: Michael K. Brawer et al., "Screening for prostatic carcinoma with prostate specific antigen," *Journal of Urology* 147 (1992), pp. 841–845. This relatively poor degree of prediction is offset by the fact that nearly 75 percent of cancers detected within the "gray zone" of PSA values between 4 and 10 are confined to the gland and thus potentially curable. Less than half of the prostate cancers detected when PSA values rise above 10 are confined to the gland. To complicate matters even more, these studies indicate some 15 percent of men above the age of sixty who had consistently normal PSA levels (less than 4) and normal rectal examinations will be found to have prostate cancer over seven years of annual screening. This observation shows that there is not a clear cutoff between what is a "normal" and an "abnormal" PSA. See Scott M. Gilbert et al., "Evidence suggesting PSA cutpoint of 2.5 ng/mL for prompting prostate biopsy: Review of 36,316 biopsies," *Urology* 65 (2005), pp. 549–553; William J. Catalona, Deborah S. Smith, David K. Ornstein, "Prostate cancer detection in men with serum PSA concentrations of 2.6 to 4.0 ng/mL and benign prostate examination," *JAMA* 277 (1997), pp. 1452–1455; Mary McNaughton Collins, David F. Ransohoff, Michael J. Barry, "Early detection of prostate cancer," *JAMA* 278 (1997), pp. 1516–1519.

Autopsy studies of men who died in accidents like car crashes show that a significant proportion had small nests of prostate cancer that hadn't been causing symptoms and in all likelihood wouldn't have contributed to any impairment during life. Overall, prostate cancer was incidentally found in between a third and a half of middle-aged or older men; see N. Breslow et al., "Latent carcinoma of prostate at autopsy in seven areas: The international agency for research on cancer, Lyons, France," *International Journal of Cancer* 20 (1977), pp. 680–688.

There is clear concern that prostate cancer may be detected by screening at a stage that would never become clinically significant but, because of detection, prompts treatment; see William J. Catalona et al., "Detection of organ-confined prostate cancer is increased through prostate-specific antigen-based screening," *JAMA* 270 (1993), pp. 948–954; Peter H. Gann, Charles H. Hennekens, Meir J. Stampfer, "A prospective evaluation of plasma prostate-specific antigen for detection of prostatic cancer," *JAMA* 273 (1995), pp. 289–294; Gerrit Draisma et al., "Lead time and overdiagnosis in prostate-specific antigen screening: Importance of methods and context," *Journal of the National Cancer Institute* (*JNCI*) 101 (2009), pp. 274–383; Ruth Etzioni et al., "Overdiagnosis due to prostate-specific antigen screening: Lessons from U.S. prostate cancer incidence trends," *JNCI* 94 (2002), pp. 981–990; Peter R. Carroll et al., "Serum prostate-specific antigen for the early detection of prostate cancer: Always, never, or only sometimes?" *Journal of Clinical Oncology* (*JCO*) 29 (2011), pp. 345–347; E. David Crawford et al., "Comorbidity and mortality results from a randomized prostate cancer screening trial," *JCO* 29 (2011), pp. 355–361; Stacy Loeb et al., "What is the true number needed to screen and treat to save a life with prostate-specific antigen testing?" *JCO* 29 (2011), pp. 464–467.

Recent studies question the current use of changes in PSA levels to predict prostate cancer; see Andrew J. Vickers et al., "An empirical evaluation of guidelines on prostate-specific antigen velocity in prostate cancer detection," *JNCI* 103 (2011), pp. 1–8; Nicholas Bakalar, "Prostate guideline causes many needless biopsies, study says," *New York Times*, February 27, 2011.

Despite these vexing issues, the death rate from prostate cancer has gradually but consistently declined since the advent of PSA screening. For example, data from Olmsted County in Minnesota, the location of the Mayo Clinic, show that age-adjusted mortality rates from prostate cancer declined 22 percent compared with the rate measured in the years before PSA testing: Manish Kohli, Donald J. Tindall, "New developments in the medical management of prostate cancer," *Mayo Clinic Proceedings* 85 (2010), pp. 77–86.

Given the controversy over the value of screening, it is not surprising that specialty organizations published different recommendations regarding PSA testing. The American Cancer Society (ACS) emphasized the need for involving men in the decision of whether to screen or not. For men who decided to be screened, the ACS recommended PSA testing for average-risk men beginning at fifty years of age. Those at higher risk, like African American men or those with a brother or father with prostate cancer diagnosed before the age of sixty-five, should begin a screening discussion at ages forty to forty-five: Andrew M. D. Wolf et al., "American Cancer Society Guideline for the early detection of prostate cancer: Update 2010," *Cancer* 60 (2010), pp. 70–98. The American Urological Association also endorsed shared decision making about risks and benefits but recommended annual screening beginning at the age forty: Kirsten L. Greene et al., "Prostate specific antigen best practice statement: 2009 update," *Journal of Urology* 182 (2009), pp. 2232–2241. The United States Preventive Services Task Force, which advises the government, concluded in 2008 that there was insufficient evidence to assess the balance of benefits and harms of prostate cancer screening in men younger than seventy-five: U.S. Preventive Services Task Force, "Screening for prostate cancer: U.S. Preventive Services Task Force Recommendation Statement," *Ann Intern Med* 149 (2008), pp. 185–191. The Canadian Task Force on Preventive Health Care recommended against screening for prostate cancer with PSA: J. W. Feightner, "Recommendations on secondary prevention of prostate cancer from the Canadian Task Force on the Periodic Health Examination," *Canadian Journal of Oncology* 4 (Suppl. 1) (1994), pp. 80–81. The American College of Physicians, an organization of internists, recommended individualizing the decision to screen after a thorough discussion with the patient: Kenneth Lin et al., "Benefits and harms of prostate-specific antigen screening for prostate cancer: An evidence update for the U.S. Preventive Services Task Force," *Ann Intern Med* 149 (2008), pp. 192–199.

Given this complexity, some researchers are developing decision aids to present data on risks and benefits of PSA screening as clearly as possible: Melissa R. Partin et al., "Randomized trial examining the effect of two prostate cancer screening educational interventions on patient knowledge, preferences, and behaviors," *JGIM* 19 (2004), pp. 835–842.

88 For the staging of prostate cancer, including the Gleason score, see Mack Roach III et al., "Staging for prostate cancer," *Cancer* 109 (2007), pp. 213–220; Sadeq Abuzallouf, Ian Dayes, Himu Lukka, "Baseline staging of newly diagnosed prostate cancer: A summary of the literature," *Journal of Urology* 171 (2004), pp. 2122–2127. A description of a prostate biopsy and ultra-

sound examination is found in Jerome Groopman, "The prostate paradox: There are new techniques for fighting the cancer: But when should we use them?" *New Yorker*, May 29, 2000.

91   Optimal therapy of prostate cancer is widely debated among medical experts. The U.S. Agency for Healthcare Research and Quality commissioned a review of treatments of prostate cancer, seeking to identify which approach might be superior in terms of either maximum cure or least side effects. A committee of nine experts, led by Dr. Timothy Wilt of the Minneapolis VA Health Care System, compared surgery, radiation, hormonal therapy, and active surveillance ("watchful waiting"). They also looked at several less common options, like cryotherapy, which quickly freezes and thaws cancer cells to destroy them. The group's analysis was guided by input from urologists, oncologists, primary care physicians, radiation therapists, and patients. The committee examined more than seven hundred published studies, assessed doctors and hospitals, patient databases, surveys, and clinical trials, weighed side effects, and evaluated survival outcomes. The conclusion was that no one treatment was superior, that all had downsides, and that fewer side effects developed among patients treated by surgeons in medical centers that performed more operations. Where the doctor stood depended largely on where he or she sat, meaning surgeons favored surgery, radiation oncologists favored radiation therapy. Notably, only a small number of doctors favored watchful waiting, although the expert panel could not discern whether this approach might be superior or inferior to the active interventions of operation and radiation.

The results of this expert analysis came as a surprise to some, since the notion that served as the basis for the review was that if specialists carefully weighed existing information, key advantages and disadvantages of the different treatment options would be identified, so-called comparative effectiveness, and a clear idea of what is "best" and for whom would become apparent. See commentary on Dr. Wilt's effort: Jenny Marder, "A user's guide to cancer treatment," *Science* 326 (2009), p. 1184.

Also of note, there were regional differences in the percentage of patients with prostate cancer who received different therapies. This was most striking with regard to watchful waiting, where about 7 percent of men in New England chose this approach versus 14 percent in the Pacific states and 13 percent in the mountain region: Agency for Healthcare Research and Quality, "Effective health care: Comparative effectiveness of therapies for clinically localized prostate cancer," *Executive Summary*, February 2008; Timothy J. Wilt et al., "Systematic review: Comparative effectiveness and harms of treatments for clinically localized prostate cancer," *Ann Intern Med* 148 (2008), pp. 435–448.

92 Matt Conlin's age and the cutoff of sixty-five years old used by the surgeon might be derived from one study indicating a survival benefit from surgery for men at or below that age: Anna Bill-Axelson et al., "Radical prostatectomy versus watchful waiting in early prostate cancer," *NEJM* 352 (2005), pp. 1977–1984. A follow-up study published in 2011 showed that the survival benefit was sustained: Anna Bill-Axelson et al., "Radical prostatectomy versus watchful waiting in early prostate cancer," NEJM 364 (2011), pp. 1708–1717; Matthew R. Smith, "Effective treatment for early-stage prostate cancer—possible, necessary, or both?" *NEJM* (editorial) 364 (2011), pp. 1770–1772.

94 Among the many studies on complications from treatment of prostate cancer, the reader may find these most relevant to the issues that men face: Shilajit D. Kundu et al., "Potency, continence and complications in 3,477 consecutive radical retropubic prostatectomies," *Journal of Urology* 172 (2004), pp. 2227–2231; David F. Penson et al., "5-year urinary and sexual outcomes after radical prostatectomy: Results from the prostate cancer outcomes study," *Journal of Urology* 173 (2005), pp. 1701–1705; Mark S. Litwin et al., "Quality of life after surgery, external beam irradiation, or brachytherapy for early-stage prostate cancer," *Cancer* 109 (2007), pp. 2239–2247; Juanita Crook et al., "Systematic overview of the evidence for brachytherapy in clinically localized prostate cancer," *CMAJ* 164 (2001), pp. 975–981; Jerry D. Slater et al., "Proton therapy for prostate cancer: The initial Loma Linda University experience," *International Journal of Radiation Oncology, Biology, Physics* 59 (2004), pp. 348–352; Michael L. Blute, "Radical prostatectomy by open or laparoscopic/robotic techniques: An issue of surgical device or surgical expertise?" *JCO* 26 (2008), pp. 2248–2249; Jim C. Hu et al., "Comparative effectiveness of minimally invasive vs. open radical prostatectomy," *JAMA* 302 (2009), pp. 1557–1564.

96 For the marked limitations of using methods like standard gamble to determine treatment preferences, see Sara J. Knight et al., "Pilot study of a utilities-based treatment decision intervention for prostate cancer patients," *Clinical Prostate Cancer* (September 2002), pp. 105–114.

Schwartz and Bergus point out that there is no standard definition of "perfect health" (*Medical Decision Making: A Physician's Guide* [Cambridge, UK: Cambridge University Press, 2008]). The rating scale method between

0 as death and 100 as perfect health is usually taken as a percentage, so that if someone was to designate a value of 50, this would be 50 percent, or 0.50. One of the major problems with the linear rating scale is that it is "arbitrary," as Schwartz and Bergus point out: "When a patient indicates that blindness should receive a value of 50, there is no behavioral interpretation for that value—it means nothing beyond 'a rating of 50.'"

In the time trade-off method, patients are told their predicted life expectancy based on actuarial data and then asked to imagine that they will spend the rest of their lives in some imperfect health state and to consider what that would be like. Then they are asked to imagine that a new treatment can restore them to perfect health but will shorten their life by a given amount. Would they take the treatment? If so, how many years are worth trading for perfect health? The trade-offs continue until the patients are indifferent between the prospect of a shorter lifetime with perfect health and their full life span with imperfect health. At that point, the duration in perfect health is divided by the duration in imperfect health and a percentage obtained; this percentage is used as the number for utility for the imperfect health state. For example, if a man has a life expectancy of seventy-eight years, and he is currently fifty-four years old, he can expect to live twenty-four more years. If he is diabetic, he is asked to imagine twenty-four years with diabetes in his current health state and then given the choice between twenty-four years with diabetes or twelve years in perfect health followed by death. He prefers twenty-four years with diabetes, so he is then offered a choice between twenty-four years with diabetes and twenty-three years in perfect health, and he prefers twenty-three years in perfect health. He is then offered a choice between twenty-four years with diabetes and twenty years in perfect health, and he prefers twenty-four years with diabetes. When he is offered twenty-four years with diabetes and twenty-two years in perfect health, he is indifferent between the two choices, finding it very difficult to say which he would prefer. His utility for diabetes is calculated as 22 divided by 24, meaning the twenty-two years in perfect health divided by his life expectancy of twenty-four years with diabetes. The utility of diabetes is 91.7. This proportion is life in the better health state divided by life expectancy in the worse health state. The time trade-off method breaks down when a person states that he or she is not willing to trade off any years of life, even though those years are lived in an imperfect health state. If that was the case, then the imperfect health state has a utility of 100 percent, meaning that it is equivalent to perfect health, which clearly it is not.

This back-and-forth assessment of time traded for perfect health is used to identify "preferences" of people *without* the imperfect health condition by asking them to imagine, in the cases of prostate cancer treatment, being impotent or incontinent. A utility number is calculated this way, and the highest utility indicates "preference." All of the pitfalls in forecasting are amplified in the setting of asking people who have no experience of the health condition to trade off time to regain "perfect health." Yet the time trade-off method is widely used in guiding clinicians; see Julia H. Hayes et al., "Active surveillance compared with initial treatment for men with low-risk prostate cancer," *JAMA* 304 (2010), pp. 2373–2380; Ian M. Thompson, Laurence Klotz, "Active surveillance for prostate cancer," *JAMA* 304 (2010), pp. 2411–2412.

To apply the standard gamble calculation for diabetes, researchers would ask a patient if she prefers living with diabetes to a treatment that results in perfect health in 90 percent of patients and death in 10 percent. Say she does not like these odds but ultimately is willing to accept a 94 percent chance of perfect health and a 6 percent chance of death. Her utility then for diabetes is 0.94. Some researchers who favor the standard gamble method point out that it incorporates the patient's risk attitude, and the odds the patient selects reflect her tolerance for risk. But there are clear difficulties with the standard gamble. A gamble involving death seems to be too "high stakes" to be reasonable for some patients. This indeed proved to be the case in trying to use the standard gamble in the setting of decisions around treatment of prostate cancer. Some patients refused to gamble and therefore would not accept any odds despite living with incontinence and impotence. This would mean that incontinence and impotence are equivalent to perfect health and have utility of 100 percent; see Sara J. Knight et al., "Pilot study of a utilities-based treatment decision intervention for prostate cancer patients," *Clinical Prostate Cancer* (September 2002), pp. 105–114.

For more detailed critiques of utility methodology, see Heather P. Lacey et al., "Are they really that happy? Exploring scale recalibration in estimates of well-being," *Health Psychology* 27 (2008), pp. 669–675; Peter A. Ubel et al., "What is perfect health to an 85-year-old? Evidence for scale recalibration in subjective health ratings, *Medical Care* 43 (2005), pp. 1054–1057; Paul Dolan, Daniel Kahneman, "Interpretations of utility and their implications for the valuation of health," *Economic Journal* 118 (2008), pp. 215–234.

Bernoulli's formula could be applied to the other patients we have met. Susan Powell, in assessing the first part of the formula on outcomes of elevated cholesterol, might ask: What kind of heart attack? Some heart attacks are minor, others lead to chronic debility with heart failure. Does the imagined heart attack lead to problems with her heart rhythm, so that she needs to take multiple medications with multiple side effects to keep her heart beating at a steady and safe pace? Is she left short of breath? Must she enter a cardiac rehabilitation program to regain her endurance? Can she return to work and spend productive days, or is she left homebound and dependent on others? Then, what kind of stroke? Does the stroke cause her arm or leg to be paralyzed or both? Is the stroke on the dominant side of her brain or the nondominant, so that there are different degrees of impairment with regard to speech and memory? Will she be unable to find and articulate the words to express herself? Does she become so forgetful that she can't remember the hymns she loves to sing each Sunday at church? How much improvement might occur after the stroke, after months of intensive physical or occupational therapy? According to Bernoulli's formula of "rational" decision making, Susan would assign a utility to each of these multiple outcomes and then multiply that number by the chance the outcome would occur. Even "simple" choices like taking a statin medication can become complex once a person begins to consider how many different outcomes could occur and their level of severity.

Jansen et al. studied unstable preferences: Sylvia J. T. Jansen et al., "Unstable preferences: A shift valuation or an effect of the elicitation procedure?" *Medical Decision Making* 20 (2000), pp. 62–71. Fifty-five breast cancer patients were evaluated before, during, and after post-op therapy. They were initially presented with a hypothetical scenario regarding radiation treatment or chemotherapy. There was a disconnect between the experienced health state and the prediction of life from the hypothetical scenario. The researchers concluded that "utilities," meaning the value that people place on different health states, are not stable but change with experience.

A similar finding, widely cited in the field of research on forecasting, was made by Peter Ubel et al., "Misimaging the unimaginable: The disability paradox in health care decision making," *Health Psychology* 24 (2005), pp. S57–S62. The "disability paradox" is the observation that people mispredict the impact that circumstances will have on their well-being and quality of life. Across a wide range of health conditions, patients typically report greater happiness and quality of life than do healthy people imagining the patients' circumstance.

Among patients with illness, misreports can be due to (1) scale recalibration, meaning that what 90 out of 100 means to one person can be something different to another; (2) conversational context, meaning patients respond differently when they know they are being surveyed as patients (this is certainly true with prostate cancer outcomes); (3) theory-driven recall bias: "I must have been less happy back then, because I think I am getting happier over time" (theory-driven recall bias comes in part from the work of Michael Ross, "Relation of implicit theories to the construction of personal histories," *Psychological Review* 96 [1989], pp. 341–357; Ross demonstrated this phenomenon in many other contexts, showing that people typically remember being less happy five years ago than they are currently, despite experiencing stable levels of happiness); (4) global judgments versus momentary moods: Despite experiencing moods rated, for example, at 5, 6, 5, 6, 7, out of 10 over the past day, the patient reports experiencing an average mood of 7 out of 10, since "7" was the most recent mood state.

There are several reasons to believe that moment-to-moment measures are more accurate than global measures. For example, when making global assessments, people place disproportionate weight on their recent moods (Daniel Kahneman et al., "When more pain is preferred to less: Adding a better end," *Psychological Science* 4 [1993], pp. 401–405). In other research, one study looked at forty-nine dialysis patients with kidney failure versus forty-nine healthy controls matched by age, race, gender, and education. Researchers gave each subject a PalmPilot program to beep at random intervals of the week and then asked them about their mood on a scale of minus 2 (very unpleasant) to 2 (very pleasant). Both groups reported experiencing positive moods significantly more often than negative moods. Despite the similarity in the moods of the kidney failure patient group versus the healthy group, neither group predicted that the other one felt the way it did. For example, when imagining they had kidney failure, healthy people predicted being in a happy mood much less frequently. This misprediction fits a pattern of healthy people underestimating the well-being of people with chronic illness or disability. Moreover, dialysis patients imagining their prior health overinflated how often they felt happy, as reflected in their assessment of their predictions for the control healthy group. We all have stereotypes in our mind of sickness and health, and these stereotypes cause us to mispredict the moods of people whose circumstances differ from our own.

Daniel Kahneman, the Nobel laureate who, with Amos Tversky, identified many cardinal cognitive biases, concluded that the fundamental paradigm of utility assessment in health is flawed. Kahneman compared assigning a single number to a patient's utility with the flawed concept in the field of physics of an ether surrounding the earth in the nineteenth century: Daniel Kahneman, "A different approach to health state valuation," special issue, *Value in Health* 12 (2009), pp. S16–S17.

97 The data given to patients on impact of side effects come from studies like Jim C. Hu et al., "Utilization and outcomes of minimally invasive radical prostatectomy," *JCO* 26 (2008), pp. 2278–2284; Wesley M. White et al., "Quality of life in men with locally advanced adenocarcinoma of the prostate: An exploratory analysis using data from the CaPSURE database," *Journal of Urology* 180 (2008), pp. 2409–2414.

There is growing literature on cognitive pitfalls in forecasting and in assigning numbers to quality of life. Gretchen Chapman, the psychologist at Rutgers, reviewed scores of studies and concluded, "Biases that affect utility assessment mean that the utilities incorporated in decision analyses often do not reflect patients' true preferences" (from D. Koehler and N. Harvey (eds.), *Blackwell Handbook of Judgment and Decision Making* [Oxford, UK: Blackwell Publishing, 2004], chapter 29, "The Psychology of Medical Decision Making," pp. 585–603). She points out that sick people need to imagine what life would be without their illness—that is, in "perfect health"—so "opening the door for the same sorts of biased predictions that affect utility valuations provided by non-patients." In that regard, Dr. Peter Ubel, formerly of the University of Michigan and now at Duke University, studied patients with kidney failure and asked them to predict life after a successful transplant, and colostomy patients who later had their colostomies reversed. The utility of better health imagined by these patients when ill did not correspond to the reality of their health state experienced later: Dylan M. Smith, Stephanie L. Brown, Peter A. Ubel, "Are subjective well-being measures any better than decision utility measures?" *Health Economics, Policy and Law* 3 (2008), pp. 85–91; Dylan M. Smith et al., "Misremembering colostomies? Former patients give lower utility ratings than do current patients," *Health Psychology* 25 (2006), pp. 688–695.

98 Daniel Gilbert, the professor of psychology at Harvard University who has extensively studied forecasting and its biases, considers Bernoulli's formula and concludes that such calculations drawn from economic decision making are "beautiful useless abstractions" since no one can reliably assign a numerical value and predict his or her level of contentment and pleasure as life changes (Daniel Gilbert, *Stumbling on Happiness* [New York: Vintage Books, 2005]). For research studies or biases in forecasting, see Daniel T. Gilbert, Timothy D. Wilson, "Prospection: Experiencing the future," *Science* 317 (2007), pp. 1351–1354; Yoav Bar-Anan, Timothy D. Wilson, "The feeling of uncertainty intensifies affective reactions," *Emotion* 9 (2009), pp. 123–127; Sarit A. Golub, Daniel T. Gilbert, "Anticipating one's troubles: The costs and

benefits of negative expectations," *Emotion* 9 (2009), pp. 277–281; Carey K. Morewedge, Daniel T. Gilbert, Timothy D. Wilson, "The least likely of times: How remembering the past biases forecasts of the future," *Psychological Science* 16 (2005), pp. 626–630; Daniel T. Gilbert, Timothy D. Wilson, "Why the brain talks to itself: Sources of error in emotional prediction," *Philosophical Transactions of the Royal Society* 364 (2009), pp. 1335–1341.

Despite these significant limitations, many treatment guidelines rely on preference calculations using time trade-off and standard gamble. And the severe flaws in the methods do not stop different therapies from being prioritized as superior or inferior or, in some settings, paid for or denied coverage: Paul Dolan, "Developing methods that really do value the 'Q' in the QALY," *Health Economics, Policy and Law* 3 (2008), pp. 69–77; Paul Dolan, "In defense of subjective well-being," *Health Economics, Policy and Law* 3 (2008), pp. 93–95. A defense of QALYs that we find unconvincing: Peter J. Neumann, "What next for QALYs?" *JAMA* (commentary) 305 (2011), pp. 1806–1807.

Some researchers are trying to develop metrics for the quality of physician decision making rather than relying on the current metrics for quality care: Karen R. Sepucha et al., "Developing instruments to measure the quality of decisions: Early results for a set of symptom-driven decisions," *Patient Education and Counseling* 73 (2008), pp. 504–510.

100 To learn more about the differences in how patients and physicians assess side effects, see Arthur S. Elstein et al., "Agreement between prostate cancer patients and their clinicians about utilities and attribute importance," *Health Expectations* 7 (2004), pp. 115–125; and Gretchen B. Chapman et al., "Prostate cancer patients' utilities for health states: How it looks depends on where you stand," *Med Decis Making* 18 (1998), pp. 278–286.

106 See note for page 91 above.

107 Barry Schwartz, a professor of psychology at Swarthmore College, noted in his book *The Paradox of Choice* (New York: Harper Perennial, 2005) that when the choice set is large, people are more likely to regret a decision that does not turn out well. They may, in his words, "stew" about the options not taken and have overinflated their expectations about the chosen option in advance. See also Schwartz, "Tyranny of choice," *Scientific American* 290 (April 2004).

109 Daniel Gilbert's experiment with Harvard undergraduates asked one very interesting question: Will people more reliably forecast their experience of

some future condition by reading a hypothetical scenario or by speaking with individuals who are similar to them and have already experienced it? In a series of such experiments, Gilbert found that reaction to reading the description of the experience did not predict how the students would experience it. But when a student spoke with another student of what it was like to experience the condition, then the prediction was more accurate: Daniel T. Gilbert et al., "The surprising power of neighborly advice," *Science* 323 (2009), pp. 1617–1619, and supplemental material online. This research prompts us to seek people who seem similar to ourselves and to listen to their tales of what it was like to undergo a treatment or experience an illness. This is a more refined approach to extracting knowledge than from random anecdotes and testimonials on the Internet.

111 Among healthy people, misprediction of life with a certain clinical condition may occur because of (1) a focusing illusion; for instance, when imagining a colostomy, people focus narrowly on the plastic pouches and the perils of wearing bathing suits at the beach without considering life domains unaffected by a colostomy; and (2) an underestimation of adaptation, in that people fail to consider how and why emotions are likely to change over time following the onset of an illness or disability.

111 For example, Peter Ubel and others studied 195 patients who had received a colostomy at the University of Michigan over the prior ten years. Approximately half of the patients surveyed had had their colostomy reversed. Across a wide range of quality-of-life and mood measures, they found no significant differences between the patients who still had colostomies and those who had their colostomies reversed. The results suggested that the effects of colostomy on overall quality of life were relatively minor. What could explain these very different answers about colostomies? Ubel and co-workers posited that people misremembered what it was like to live with a colostomy. This kind of recall bias can be very powerful; see Laura J. Damschroder, Brian J. Zikmund-Fisher, Peter A. Ubel, "Considering adaptation in preference elicitations," *Health Psychology* 27 (2008), pp. 394–399; Dylan M. Smith et al., "Misremembering colostomies? Former patients give lower utility ratings than do current patients," *Health Psychology* 25 (2006), pp. 688–695.

111 When imagining unfamiliar circumstances, people focus narrowly on the most obvious difference between those circumstances and their current circumstances and thereby mispredict the emotional impact of the change in circumstances. This is termed a "focusing illusion." College students living

in the Midwest reported levels of happiness similar to levels of those living in Southern California. Yet students in both locations predict that life would be better in California than in the Midwest. Why? People focus narrowly on the better climate in Southern California, and students downplay all the nonweather-related things that make college life enjoyable or unenjoyable. They seem to forget that happiness in college depends more on the kinds of friends you hang out with than on whether you can hang out with them in consistently sunny weather. See David A. Schkade, Daniel Kahneman, "Does living in California make people happy? A focusing illusion in judgments of life satisfaction," *Psychological Science* 9 (1998), pp. 340–346; Daniel Kahneman et al., "Would you be happier if you were richer? A focusing illusion," *Science* 312 (2006), pp. 1908–1910. In medicine, focusing illusions could contribute to the disability paradox because healthy people overestimate the emotional impact of a chronic illness or disability by focusing narrowly on those domains of their life that are influenced by illness and disability, imagining being much less happy than they would really be.

111 Insightful books on resilience and adaptation: Richard M. Cohen, *Blindsided: Lifting a Life Above Illness* (HarperCollins, 2004); *Strong at the Broken Places: Voices of Illness, a Chorus of Hope* (HarperCollins, 2008).

111 Dana Jennings further reflected: "I've trudged through Stage 3 prostate cancer and its treatment in good shape. Nearly two years after learning I had cancer, I'm an active fifty-two-year-old, I exercise regularly, my blood tests are where they need to be, and my oncologist wants to see me only twice a year.

"But there is one side effect of my treatment that has proved especially stubborn: erectile dysfunction.

"Prostate cancer and its treatment strike men where they live, often causing impotence and incontinence. (My bladder control gradually returned. But I can still be caught off guard by the stray sneaky sneeze.)

"Where does that leave a man who has erectile dysfunction? . . . True manhood is about love and kindness. It's about responsibility and honor, about working hard and raising your children the best way you know how, with love, respect, and discipline."

CHAPTER 6: AUTONOMY AND COPING

115 Julie's feelings about the "best of the best" as a factor in her choice: Paul Slovic, Ellen Peters, Melissa L. Finucane, Donald G. MacGregor, "Affect, risk, and decision making," *Health Psychology* 24 (2005), pp. S35–S40. This

work focuses on the powerful pull of intuition and emotions that can influence the process of decision making.

115 Patients may, as Julie Brody did, go through their "Rolodex," contacting people who are "in the know" to identify that one doctor who seems to stand above all the rest. Others may consult published lists centered around their city, like those in *New York* magazine or *Boston* magazine. With the advent of Internet rating sites for everything from chefs to housepainters, there has been a proliferation of popular ratings of physicians on the Web. Many of these profiles are derived from testimonials and often have no filter. Some of the vignettes on the Internet may be accurate, while other stories reflect the opinions of particular patients who were delighted with their physicians or became alienated, each for reasons that may not be relevant to you.

115 Mary Frances Luce at Duke University summarized her own work and the work of several other researchers in decision making and coping: Mary Frances Luce, "Decision making as coping," *Health Psychology* 24 (2005), pp. S23–S28. There is extensive literature on the psychology of coping with illness. Some of the articles most relevant to Julie Brody's concerns about finding "the best of the best" and understanding the elements of her relationship with her doctor that foster coping include Susan Folkman, "Personal control and stress and coping processes: A theoretical analysis," *Journal of Personality and Social Psychology* 46 (1984), pp. 839–852; and Amy B. Goldring et al., "Impact of health beliefs, quality of life, and the physician-patient relationship on the treatment intentions of inflammatory bowel disease patients," *Health Psychology* 21 (2002), pp. 219–228. Research specific to coping with breast cancer includes Vicki S. Helgeson, Pamela Snyder, Howard Seltman, "Psychological and physical adjustment to breast cancer over 4 years: Identifying distinct trajectories of change," *Health Psychology* 23 (2004), pp. 3–15; Sharon R. Sears, Annette L. Stanton, Sharon Daoff-Burg, "The yellow brick road and the emerald city: Benefit finding, positive reappraisal coping, and posttraumatic growth in women with early-stage breast cancer," *Health Psychology* 22 (2003), pp. 487–497; and Lesley F. Degner et al., "Information needs and decisional preferences in women with breast cancer," *JAMA* 277 (1997), pp. 1485–1492.

115 Decisional conflict is a major area of study in psychology. For a seminal paper, see Amos Tversky, Eldar Shafir, "Choice under conflict: The dynamics of deferred decision," *Psychological Science* 3 (1992), pp. 358–361. Some relevant articles on this topic in patient choice include France Legare et al.,

"The effect of decision aids on the agreement between women's and physicians' decisional conflict about hormone replacement therapy," *Patient Education and Counseling* 50 (2003), pp. 211–221; Annie LeBlanc, David A. Kenny, Annette M. O'Connor, France Legare, "Decisional conflict in patients and their physicians: A dyadic approach to shared decision making," *Medical Decision Making* 29 (2009), pp. 61–68; Annette M. O'Connor et al., "Do patient decision aids meet effectiveness criteria of the International Patient Decision Aid Standards Collaboration? A systematic review and meta-analysis," *Medical Decision Making* 27 (2007), pp. 554–574; and France Legare et al., "Are you SURE? Assessing patient decisional conflict with a 4-item screening test," *Canadian Family Physician* 56 (2010), pp. E308–E314.

117 The paradigm of hot/cold decision making is presented in George Loewenstein, "Hot-cold empathy gaps and medical decision making," *Health Psychology* 24 (2005), pp. S49–S56. The potential benefit of anticipatory regret is to be found in Terry Connolly and Jochen Reb, "Regret in cancer-related decisions," *Health Psychology* 24 (2005), pp. S29–S34.

118 The 2007 survey of how patients choose their doctors is found in Ha T. Tu, Johanna R. Lauer, "Word of mouth and physician referrals still drive health care provider choice," *HSC Research Brief* (Center for Studying Health System Change, Washington, DC) 9 (December 2008). The failure of quality metrics and physician report cards to encompass physician judgment is powerfully presented in Danielle Ofri, "Quality measures and the individual physician," *NEJM* 363 (2010), pp. 606–607. An analytical study from the RAND Corporation highlighting the deficiencies of rating systems based on cost efficiency is found in John L. Adams, Ateev Mehrotra, J. William Thomas, Elizabeth A. McGlynn, "Physician cost profiling: Reliability and risk of misclassification," *NEJM* 362 (2010), pp. 1014–1021. Also see Janet Colwell, "Should doctors worry about online ratings?" *ACP Internist* 30 (2010), pp. 1, 16. Despite such caveats, there is considerable effort to make such metrics primary in patient choices: Michelle Andrews, "Insurers and ratings groups post information to help patients choose doctors," *Washington Post*, August 3, 2010. In a notable article in the *Sunday New York Times* titled "Metric Mania," a mathematician raised the valid concern that society is too often trying to measure dimensions of experience that are not amenable to calculation: John Allen Paulos, "Metric mania," *New York Times Magazine*, May 16, 2010. Also see Gary Wolf, "The data-driven life: Tech-

nology has made it feasible not only to measure our most basic habits but also to evaluate them: Does measuring what we eat or how much we sleep or how often we do the dishes change how we think about ourselves?" *New York Times Magazine*, May 2, 2010.

118 Choosing a physician in some ways has similarities to choosing a companion with whom you can share confidences and trust that your interests are paramount. A related example of metrics in online dating and how they fall short of key elements in relationships is wonderfully presented by Dan Ariely, *The Upside of Irrationality: The Unexpected Benefits of Defying Logic at Work and at Home* (New York: HarperCollins, 2010), and Courtney Humphries, "Data mining the heart: How do we choose a mate? What scientists are learning from online dating," *Boston Sunday Globe*, August 22, 2010.

118 A number of states, including ours, have begun to post report cards on the Internet on physicians. The validity of these ratings is highly questionable. For example, an experienced pediatrician who works in a poor neighborhood in Boston was given low marks because she did not fulfill several "quality measures" needed to prove her worth. Many of these measures were not meaningful in the context of patient care, and the state agency that ranked her made no effort to assess the clinical outcomes of the children in her practice. The Massachusetts Medical Society featured her plight as an example of the capriciousness of some of the rankings: Tom Walsh, "Physicians cite continuing problems with fourth year of GIC tiering," *Vital Signs* 14 (April 2009), http://www.massmed.org/AM/Template.cfm?Section=Home 6&TEMPLATE=/CM/ContentDisplay.cfm&CONTENTID=29032; Emily Berry, "Challenging your rating: You don't have to accept what the health plan says," *American Medical News* 52, no. 10 (2009), posted online March 23, 2009, http://www.ama-assn.org/amednews/2009/03/23/bisa 0323.htm. Also see failure of quality measures to improve patient health: NICE-SUGAR Study Investigators, "Intensive versus conventional glucose control in critically ill patients," *NEJM* 360 (2009), pp. 1283–1297; Silvo E. Inzucchi, Mark D. Siegel, "Glucose control in the ICU: How tight is too tight?" *NEJM* 360 (2009), pp. 1346–1349; Bengt C. Fellstrom et al., "Rosuvastatin and cardiovascular events in patients undergoing hemodialysis," *NEJM* 360 (2009), pp. 1395–1407; Robert G. Dluhy, Graham T. McMahon, "Intensive glycemic control in the ACCORD and ADVANCE trials," *NEJM* 358 (2008), pp. 2630–2633; William T. Cefalu, "Glycemic targets

and cardiovascular disease," *NEJM* 358(2008), pp. 2633–2635; Action to Control Cardiovascular Risk in Diabetes Study Group, "Effects of intensive glucose lowering in type 2 diabetes," *NEJM* 358 (2008), pp. 2545–2559; ADVANCE Collaborative Group, "Intensive blood glucose control and vascular outcomes in patients with type 2 diabetes," *NEJM* 358 (2008), pp. 2560–2572; Gregg C. Fonarow et al., "Association between performance measures and clinical outcomes for patients hospitalized with heart failure," *JAMA* 297 (2007), pp. 61–70; Timothy Bhattacharyya et al., "Measuring the report card: The validity of pay-for-performance metrics in orthopedic surgery," *Health Affairs* 28 (2009), pp. 526–532. Also see Jerome Groopman, Pamela Hartzband, "Why 'quality' care is dangerous," *Wall Street Journal*, April 8, 2009; Jerome Groopman, Pamela Hartzband, "Sorting fact from fiction on health care," *Wall Street Journal*, August 31, 2009.

119 Certain quantitative measures are valuable for a patient to consult. The number of cases a surgeon has performed often correlates with his or her expertise. This is because there is a "learning curve" in performing a certain procedure. Similarly, safety data can be very informative, like a hospital's track record of serious complications; this has been shown accurate in assessing potentially preventable infections that occur when inserting a catheter into a vein. But beyond safety there is great difficulty in assessing "quality care" because of the complexity and severity of many clinical conditions. For example, a cardiologist who chooses to treat only those with mild heart disease will have better outcomes, and a better report card, than another who takes on the difficult, challenging cases. Such complex patients require more of a doctor's time and incur significantly more costs. Indeed, a study from the Brigham and Women's Hospital showed that some cardiologists in Boston were avoiding caring for very sick and complicated patients with heart disease because of fear that their report cards would look bad; see Frederick S. Resnic, Frederick G. P. Welt, "The public health hazards of risk avoidance associated with public reporting of risk-adjusted outcomes in coronary intervention," *Journal of the American College of Cardiology* 53 (2009), pp. 825–830. And for similar findings in California, see Cheryl L. Damberg et al., "Taking stock of pay-for-performance: A candid assessment from the front lines," *Health Affairs* 28 (2009), pp. 517–525. Cost is also a major factor in physician ratings: Cheaper care is often rated more highly. But a study of major California hospitals showed that the more money spent on a patient with heart failure, the more likely he or she was

to survive: Michael K. Ong et al., "Looking forward, looking back: Assessing variations in hospital resource use and outcomes for elderly patients with heart failure," *Circulation Cardiovascular Quality and Outcomes* 2 (2009), pp. 548–557.

121 The debate about radiation for Julie centered on issues of both quality of life and long-term survival. Before the advent of modern radiation techniques, radiation was routinely recommended for all women undergoing mastectomy who had cancer that had spread to the lymph nodes. Its use declined sharply following many reports of an adverse impact, both side effects with damage to the heart and unclear benefit with regard to survival. The risk to the heart has greatly reduced with ways to more accurately focus the beam and avoid damaging cardiac tissue. This then shifted the debate to how radiation may or may not help women like Julie Brody. Women at high risk for recurrent breast cancer often have the tumor recur locally, at the site of mastectomy and where the lymph nodes were excised. Women with such "local recurrence" not only suffer from the cancer growing on their chest, but also have a higher rate of metastasis appearing in bone, liver, and lung. A clinical trial in British Columbia of women at high risk for return of the breast cancer in the local area where the breast and lymph nodes were removed showed that there was a significant benefit in overall survival when radiation was given after mastectomy. We have seen how such data can be presented to look more impressive, like using a relative reduction in risk that can appear to be very large while in reality it is very minor. So let's assess for results in detail, looking not at relative benefit but at absolute benefit. The absolute reduction in mortality was 11 percent in women with one to three positive nodes and 7 percent in those with more than four nodes: Joseph Ragaz et al., "Locoregional radiation therapy in patients with high-risk breast cancer receiving adjuvant chemotherapy: 20-year results of the British Columbia randomized trial," *JNCI* 97 (2005), p. 116–126. Furthermore, a so-called meta-analysis from the Early Breast Cancer Trialists' Collaborative Group looked at forty-six randomized trials involving over twenty-three thousand patients. In the group of more than eighty-five hundred women who had cancer in lymph nodes and received radiation after mastectomy, the improvement in survival was highly significant at sixteen years, with six out of one hundred *more* women dying from the tumor who had *not* received radiation compared with those who had: Early Breast Cancer Trialists' Collaborative Group, "Effects of radiotherapy and of differences in the

extent of surgery for early breast cancer on local recurrence and 15-year survival: An overview of the randomized trials," *Lancet* 366 (2005), pp. 2087–2106. In Denmark, the Breast Cancer Cooperative Group studied over seventeen thousand premenopausal women like Julie Brody, who had cancer that had spread to the lymph nodes or other worrisome findings. Radiation therapy after mastectomy and chemotherapy, with a ten-year follow-up, showed that only 9 percent who received radiation had the tumor reappear on the chest wall versus 32 percent who had not received radiation. Furthermore, the disease did not come back (so-called disease-free survival) in 48 percent of those who received radiation versus 35.4 percent of those who did not. Overall survival also was quite different—54 percent in the radiation group lived versus 45 percent without radiation. See Marie Overgaard et al., "Postoperative radiotherapy in high-risk premenopausal women with breast cancer who received adjuvant chemotherapy," *NEJM* 337 (1997), pp. 949–955. These findings were in concert with the studies from British Columbia, where 50 percent of women with cancer in their lymph nodes who had not entered menopause and received radiation therapy after mastectomy were free of cancer and alive at fifteen years, versus 33 percent of women who were free of cancer if they did not receive radiation. There was also a trend toward improved overall survival of 54 percent versus 46 percent in the group not receiving radiation. At twenty years, there was an overall survival benefit of 47 percent versus 37 percent; in those with one to three positive lymph nodes, there was 7 percent absolute survival (57 percent versus 50 percent).

121 The criticism of these results came largely from surgeons, who noted that in studies done in the United States, where more lymph nodes were removed from women at the time of mastectomy, the failure rate in terms of the tumor returning at the site of the surgery was much lower than in either British Columbia or Denmark. This informed the discussion when Julie Brody's oncologist presented her case at the clinical conference. Surgeons there, including the one who operated on Brody, argued that with a more complete operation, most of the patients with one to three positive lymph nodes would actually have been found to have four more positive nodes, and this accounted for the apparent survival benefit in this group. "Her prognosis is still quite good without the radiation, and I removed every node that needed to be removed," her surgeon stated.

121 The debate continues. And even among expert committees, there are differences in guidelines. The National Comprehensive Cancer Network pub-

lished recommendations that radiation should be "strongly considered" in women like Julie Brody with one to three positive nodes (http://www.nccn .org/professionals/physician_gls/f_guidelines.asp). But the American Society of Clinical Oncology, which includes specialists across the field of cancer treatment such as medical oncologists, radiation therapists, and surgeons, recommended radiation only in patients with four or more positive nodes. See Abram Recht et al., "Postmastectomy radiotherapy: Guidelines of the American Society of Clinical Oncology," *JCO* 19 (2001), pp. 1539–1569. Similar guidelines were published in Canada: Pauline T. Truong et al., "Clinical practice guidelines for the care and treatment of breast cancer: 16. locoregional post-mastectomy radiotherapy," *CMAJ* 170 (2004), pp. 1263–1273. The year that Julie was diagnosed, an editorial about radiation therapy for women like her appeared in the *Journal of Clinical Oncology:* Lawrence B. Marks et al., "One to three versus four or more positive nodes and postmastectomy radiotherapy: Time to end the debate," *JCO* 26 (2008), pp. 2075–2077. These specialists argued that all patients with one to three positive nodes should be referred to a radiation oncologist for a "thoughtful discussion of the benefits and risks of treatment so that they make an informed decision."

123 The study of Canadian women and how much control they want in decision making: Lesley F. Degner et al., "Information needs and decisional preferences in women with breast cancer," *JAMA* 277 (1997), pp. 1485–1492. Also see differences in desire for control among patients with lung or colorectal cancer: Nancy L. Keating et al., "Cancer patients' roles in treatment decisions: Do characteristics of the decision influence roles?" *JCO* 28 (2010), pp. 4364–4370.

124 The discovery and biological functions of the BRCA genes: Yoshio Miki et al., "A strong candidate for the breast and ovarian cancer susceptibility gene BRCA1," *Science* 266 (1994), pp. 66–71; Richard Wooster et al., "Identification of the breast cancer susceptibility gene BRCA2," *Nature* 378 (1995), pp. 789–792; Ashok R. Venkitaraman, "Cancer susceptibility and the functions of BRCA1 and BRCA2," *Cell* 108 (2002), pp. 171–182.

127 Choices related to being tested for BRCA mutation and which preventive measures are selected by women: Marc D. Schwartz et al., "Decision making and decision support for hereditary breast-ovarian cancer susceptibility," *Health Psychology* (2005), pp. S78–S84; Thomas Goetz, *The Decision Tree: Taking Control of Your Health in the New Era of Personalized Medicine* (New York: Rodale Books, 2010); David K. Payne et al., "Women's regrets after

bilateral prophylactic mastectomy," *Annals of Surgical Oncology* 7 (2000), pp. 150–154; Susan M. Domchek et al., "Association of risk-reducing surgery in BRCA1 or BRCA2 mutation carriers with cancer risk and mortality," *JAMA* 304 (2010), pp. 967–975; Laura Esserman, Virginia Kaklamani, "Lessons learned from genetic testing," *JAMA* 304 (2010), pp. 1011–1012; Marc D. Schwartz et al., "Utilization of BRCA1/BRCA2 mutation testing in newly diagnosed breast cancer patients," *Cancer Epidemiology, Biomarkers & Prevention* 14 (2005), pp. 1003–1007; Beth N. Peshkin et al., "Utilization of breast cancer screening in a clinically based sample of women after BRCA1/2 testing," *Cancer Epidemiology, Biomarkers & Prevention* 11 (2002), pp. 1115–1118; Lisa J. Herrinton et al., "Efficacy of prophylactic mastectomy in women with unilateral breast cancer: A cancer research network project," *JCO* 23 (2005), pp. 4275–4286; Jose G. Guillem et al., "ASCO/SSO review of current role of risk-reducing surgery in common hereditary cancer syndromes," *JCO* 24 (2006), pp. 4642–4660; Marielle S. van Roosmalen et al., "Randomized trial of a shared decision-making intervention consisting of trade-offs and individualized treatment information for BRCA1/2 mutation carriers," *JCO* 22 (2004), pp. 3293–3301; Lauren Scheuer et al., "Outcome of preventive surgery and screening for breast and ovarian cancer in BRCA mutation carriers," *JCO* 20 (2002), pp. 1260–1268.

127 The data we cite on different decisions about mastectomy and oophorectomy among BRCA positive women with or without cancer: Jeffrey R. Botkin et al., "Genetic testing for a BRCA1 mutation: Prophylactic surgery and screening behavior in women 2 years post testing," *American Journal of Medical Genetics* 118A (2003), pp. 201–209; E. J. Meijers-Heijboer et al., "Presymptomatic DNA testing and prophylactic surgery in families with a BRCA1 or BRCA2 mutation," *Lancet* 355 (2000), pp. 2015–2020; Marc D. Schwartz et al., "Bilateral prophylactic oophorectomy and ovarian cancer screening following BRCA1/BRCA2 mutation testing," *JCO* 21 (2003), pp. 4034–4041; Marc D. Schwartz et al., "Impact of BRCA1/BRCA2 counseling and testing on newly diagnosed breast cancer patients," *JCO* 22 (2004), pp. 1823–1829; Caryn Lerman et al., "Prophylactic surgery decisions and surveillance practices one year following BRCA1/2 testing," *Preventive Medicine* 31 (2000), pp. 75–80; Theresa M. Marteau, Caryn Lerman, "Genetic risk and behavioural change," *British Medical Journal* 322 (2001), pp. 1056–1059; Caryn Lerman, Robert T. Croyle, "Emotional and behavioral responses to genetic testing for susceptibility to cancer," *Oncology* 10 (1996), pp. 191–195; Kelly A. Metcalfe et al., "International variation in rates of

uptake of preventive options in BRCA1 and BRCA2 mutation carriers," *International Journal of Cancer* 122 (2008), p. 2017–2022; Elizabeth M. Kaufman et al., "Development of an interactive decision aid for female BRCA1/BRCA2 carriers," *Journal of Genetic Counseling* 12 (2003), pp. 109–129.

127 BRCA testing is the leading edge of genetic testing. In 2000, the human genome was deciphered, the DNA sequence of our twenty thousand expressed genes. The media heralded this achievement as unveiling "the code of life," a detailed blueprint that reveals how each of us is designed. The DNA code was made publicly available, posted on the Internet, by government scientists. At the same time, biotech companies announced that they would offer, for a fee, a personal profile of your genes, providing information on your predisposition for a wide variety of diseases. A heated debated ensued among scientists, ethicists, psychologists, and clinicians. How much do people want to know about the odds of a future malady? What can they do with this information? The question of whether to be tested or not, and the consequences of the knowledge, centers on loss aversion. Recall that we experience loss more profoundly than gain, and this causes many people to focus on the side effects of the choice rather than its potential benefits. The side effects in learning that you have a genetic predisposition to a disease are primarily emotional: anxiety, fear, frustration, and worry, not only about yourself but about your siblings and your children. These negative emotions are compounded when there currently is little to do about lowering the chances of the future malady, as is the case with Alzheimer's disease. Some other people seek information on risk, believing this will help them set priorities in life or prompt them to enter a research study and contribute to science. See Steven Pinker, "My genome, my self," *New York Times Magazine*, January 11, 2009; Francis S. Collin, *The Language of Life: DNA and the Revolution in Personalized Medicine* (New York: HarperCollins, 2010).

129 Hodgkin's lymphoma is one of the most studied cancers, but only within the past decade has it become clear that the malignancy arises from B lymphocytes and may be related in some cases to Epstein-Barr virus infection; see Ralf Küppers, "The biology of Hodgkin's lymphoma," *Nature Reviews Cancer* 9 (2009), pp. 15–27. Therapy of advanced Hodgkin's lymphoma in the United States, Europe, and Israel is detailed in Sandra J. Horning, "Risk, cure and complications in advanced Hodgkin disease," *Hematology* 2007, pp. 197–203; Peter J. Hoskin et al., "Randomized comparison of the Stanford V regimen and ABVD in the treatment of advanced Hodgkin's lymphoma:

United Kingdom National Cancer Research Institute Lymphoma Group Study ISRCTN 64141244," *JCO* 27 (2009), pp. 5390–5396; Eldad J. Dann et al., "Risk-adapted BEACOPP regimen can reduce the cumulative dose of chemotherapy for standard and high-risk Hodgkin lymphoma with no impairment of outcome," *Blood* 109 (2007), pp. 905–909.

131 The history of progress in treatment of Hodgkin's lymphoma is described in Siddhartha Mukherjee, *The Emperor of All Maladies: A Biography of Cancer* (New York: Charles Scribner's Sons, 2010).

134 The issue of patient autonomy is addressed in depth in Carl E. Schneider, *The Practice of Autonomy: Patients, Doctors, and Medical Decisions* (New York: Oxford University Press, 1998). The actress Jill Clayburgh died in 2010. After her death, it became known that she had had chronic lymphocytic leukemia for many years and had kept the diagnosis secret so as not to limit her career.

CHAPTER 7: DECISION ANALYSIS MEETS REALITY

140 The development of cancers like chronic lymphocytic leukemia and aggressive non-Hodgkin's lymphoma following an autoimmune muscle disease and its treatment is well described in the medical literature; see Ola Landgren et al., "Acquired immune-related and inflammatory conditions and subsequent chronic lymphocytic leukaemia," *British Journal of Haematology* 139 (2007), pp. 791–798; A. Créange et al., "Inflammatory neuromuscular disorders associated with chronic lymphoid leukemia: Evidence for clonal B cells within muscle and nerve," *Journal of the Neurological Sciences* 137 (1996), p. 35–41; Takao Endo et al., "Polymyositis-dermatomyositis and non-Hodgkin's lymphoma," *Internal Medicine* 32 (1993), pp. 487–489; László Váróczy et al., "Malignant lymphoma-associated autoimmune disease: A descriptive epidemiological study," *Rheumatology International* 22 (2002), pp. 233–237; Whon-Ho Chow et al., "Cancer risk following polymyositis and dermatomyositis: A nationwide cohort study in Denmark," *Cancer Causes and Control* 6 (1995), pp. 9–13; R. J. Evans, H. H. B. Hilton, "Polymyositis associated with acute monocytic leukemia: Case report and review of the literature," *CMAJ* 91 (1964), pp. 1272–1275; Catherine L. Hill et al., "Frequency of specific cancer types in dermatomyositis and polymyositis: A population-based study," *Lancet* 357 (2001), pp. 96–100.

144 Although chronic lymphocytic leukemia is a very common blood disorder, there is still debate among experts about when it is optimal to initiate treatment and what that treatment should be; key factors in these decisions include the rate of rise in the white count and the presence or absence of prognostic molecular markers like ZAP-70, CD38, and unmutated immunoglobulin Bh genes. In general, blood counts are performed at three-month intervals along with a physical examination. Many hematologists track the rate of increase in blood lymphocyte count as well as any new symptoms like weight loss, fever, or bleeding. Clinical studies show that survival of patients with a blood lymphocyte doubling time shorter than twelve months is significantly less than those with longer doubling times. Some clinicians decide to begin treatment in this setting, although others do not treat based on the doubling time alone. In addition, the absolute level of blood lymphocyte count needs to be considered, since doubling of the count from 10,000 to 20,000 in less than twelve months in a patient who is at an early stage of disease and free of symptoms does not have the same significance as a doubling of the count from 75,000 to 150,000; see Nicholas Chorazzi, Kanti R. Rai, M. Ferrarini, "Mechanisms of disease: Chronic lymphocytic leukemia," *NEJM* 352 (2005), pp. 804–815; Thorsten Zenz et al., "From pathogenesis to treatment of chronic lymphocytic leukaemia," *Nature Reviews Cancer* 10 (2010), pp. 37–50; John G. Gribben, "How I treat CLL up front," *Blood* 115 (2010), pp. 187–197; Stefano Molica, Antonio Alberti, "Prognostic value of lymphocyte doubling time in chronic lymphocytic leukemia," *Cancer* 60 (1987), pp. 2712–2716; Emili Monserrat et al., "Lymphocyte doubling time in chronic lymphocytic leukaemia: Analysis of its prognostic significance," *British Journal of Haematology* 62 (1986), pp. 567–575; Michael Hallek et al., "Guidelines for the diagnosis and treatment of chronic lymphocytic leukemia: A report from the International Workshop on Chronic Lymphocytic Leukemia updating the National Cancer Institute—Working Group 1996 guidelines," *Blood* 111 (2008), pp. 5446–5456.

145 Paul Peterson's chronic lymphocytic leukemia became resistant to standard treatment regimens. He faced the option of receiving more chemotherapy that might control the leukemia for a relatively short duration of time (usually months) or undergoing bone marrow transplantation. The clinical issues involved in making the choices are reviewed in Emili Montserrat et al., "How I treat refractory CLL," *Blood* 107 (2006), pp. 1276–1283.

147 The field of decision analysis was established in the 1950s. A now classical publication by John von Neumann and Oskar Morgenstern (*Theory of Games and Economic Behavior*, 2nd ed. [Princeton, NJ: Princeton University Press, 1947]) presented a normative model with rational decision making based on a set of axioms. The model was influenced by game theory and posited a so-called rational actor who applies Bernoulli's formula for maximizing expected utility. Traditional decision analysis in medicine provides a series of decision trees to structure the choice, with defined probabilities for each outcome and patient values, typically using the methods of time trade-off or standard gamble. See Stephen G. Pauker, Jerome P. Kassirer, "Decision analysis," *NEJM* 316 (1987), pp. 250–258; Gary Naglie et al., "Primer on medical decision analysis: Estimating probabilities and utilities," *Medical Decision Making* 136 (1997), pp. 136–141; Thomas Goetz, *The Decision Tree: Taking Control of Your Health in the New Era of Personalized Medicine* (New York: Rodale Books, 2010).

149 We have discussed in detail the complexity of forecasting in chapters 3 and 5. Please see endnotes for detailed references. A lively and engaging popular book by an expert in the field is Daniel Gilbert's *Stumbling on Happiness* (New York: Vintage Books, 2007). Gilbert concludes: "Yes, we *should* make choices by multiplying probabilities and utilities, but how can we possibly do this if we can't estimate those utilities beforehand? The same objective circumstances give rise to a remarkably wide variety of subjective experiences, and thus it is very difficult to predict our subjective experiences from foreknowledge of our objective circumstances. . . . The simple lawful relationships that bind numbers to numbers and words to words do not bind objective events to emotional experiences."

CHAPTER 8: END OF LIFE

153 President's Commission for the Study of Ethical Problems in Medicine and Biomedical and Behavioral Research, "Deciding to forgo life-sustaining treatment," Library of Congress card number 83-600503, March 1983; this report can be accessed via http://bioethics.georgetown.edu/pcbe/reports/past_commissions/deciding_to_forgo_tx.pdf.

154 Cancer of the biliary tract is often incurable, and survival is measured in months to years. Occasionally there are dramatic remissions, like the one that Mary Quinn experienced. See Jerome Groopman, *The Anatomy of Hope: How People Prevail in the Face of Illness* (New York: Random House,

2004), for a similar narrative of a physician who faced choices after a diagnosis of biliary cancer.

157 The SUPPORT study is found in SUPPORT Principal Investigators, "A controlled trial to improve care for seriously ill hospitalized patients: The study to understand prognoses and preferences for outcomes and risks of treatments (SUPPORT)," *JAMA* 274 (1995), pp. 1591–1598.

158 The finding that advance directives in the SUPPORT study were not consistently informative is Christina M. Puchalski et al., "Patients who want their family and physician to make resuscitation decisions for them: Observations from SUPPORT and HELP," *Journal of the American Geriatrics Society* 48 (2000), pp. S84–S90. The research from Dr. Terri Fried of Yale University on how preference is changing: Terri R. Fried et al., "Inconsistency over time in the preferences of older persons with advanced illness for life-sustaining treatment," *Journal of the American Geriatrics Society* 55 (2007), pp. 1007–1014. Also see Terri R. Fried et al., "Prospective study of health status preferences and changes in preferences over time in older adults," *Archives of Internal Medicine* 166 (2006), pp. 890–895. The article by Dr. Rebecca Sudore with Dr. Fried is found in Rebecca L. Sudore, Terri R. Fried, "Redefining the 'planning' in advance care planning: Preparing for end-of-life decision making," *Ann Intern Med* 153 (2010), pp. 256–261. Also see Rebecca L. Sudore, Dean Schillinger, Sara J, Knight, Terri R. Fried, "Uncertainty about advance care planning treatment preferences among diverse older adults," *Journal of Health Communication* 15 (Suppl. 2) (2010), pp. 159–171.

159 The commentary by Dr. Muriel Gillick is in Muriel R. Gillick, "Reversing the code status of advance directives?" *NEJM* 362 (2010), pp. 1239–1240. This was in response to an outlier study in the same issue of the *New England Journal of Medicine*: Maria J. Silveira, Scott Y. H. Kim, Kenneth M. Langa, "Advance directives and outcomes of surrogate decision making before death," *NEJM* 362 (2010), pp. 1211–1218.

159 We have discussed the difficulty in forecasting preferences under circumstances that have not yet been experienced. In addition to the studies cited in chapters 3 and 5, see Jodi Halpern, Robert M. Arnold, "Affective forecasting: An unrecognized challenge in making serious health decisions," *JGIM* 23 (2008), pp. 1708–1712; Peter H. Ditto et al., "Context changes choices: A prospective study of the effects of hospitalization on life-sustaining treatment preferences," *Medical Decision Making* 26 (2006), pp. 313–322; Peter

H. Ditto, Nikki A. Hawkins, "Advance directives and cancer decision making near the end of life," *Health Psychology* 24 (Suppl. 4) (2005), pp. S63–S70.

166 The research assessing early introduction of palliative care in patients with lung cancer is in Jennifer S. Temel et al., "Early palliative care for patients with metastatic non-small-cell lung cancer," *NEJM* 363 (2010), pp. 733–742. The accompanying editorial by Drs. Kelley and Meier is in Amy S. Kelley, Diane E. Meier, "Palliative Care: A shifting paradigm," *NEJM* 363 (2010), pp. 781–782.

167 On the difficulty in having conversations around end-of-life wishes, see Timothy E. Quill, "Initiating end-of-life discussions with seriously ill patients: Addressing the 'elephant in the room,'" *JAMA* 284 (2000), pp. 2502–2507; Stephen J. McPhee et al., "Finding our way: Perspectives on care at the close of life," *JAMA* 284 (2000), pp. 2512–2513.

182 The collection of narratives from bereaved family members in Connecticut is in Terri R. Fried, John R. O'Leary, "Using the experience of bereaved caregivers to inform patient- and caregiver-centered advance care planning," *JGIM* 23 (2008), pp. 1602–1607.

183 The effort to have physicians write specific orders about life-sustaining treatments in the patient chart at admission to hospital: Diane E. Meier, Larry Beresford, "POLST offers next stage in honoring patient preferences," *Journal of Palliative Medicine* 12 (2009), pp. 291–295; Laura Landro, "New efforts to simplify end-of-life care wishes," *Wall Street Journal*, March 15, 2011.

CHAPTER 9: WHEN THE PATIENT CAN'T DECIDE

185 The study on hospitalized patients unable to decide for themselves: Vanessa Raymont et al., "Prevalence of mental incapacity in medical inpatients and associated risk factors: Cross-sectional study," *Lancet* 364 (2004), pp. 1421–1427. Also see Jason H. T. Karlawish, "Competency in the age of assessment," *Lancet* 364 (2004), pp. 1383–1384; Shaun T. O'Keeffe, "Mental capacity of inpatients," *Lancet* 365 (2005), pp. 568–569.

188 For the story of the discovery of hepatitis B, see "The Nobel Prize in Physiology or Medicine 1976," Baruch S. Blumberg, Autobiography, http://nobelprize.org/nobel_prizes/medicine/laureates/1976/blumberg-autobio.html.

189 Hepatitis B treatment and liver transplantation: Robert P. Perrillo, Andrew L. Mason, "Hepatitis B and liver transplantation: Problems and promises,"

NEJM 329 (1993), pp. 1885–1887; Morris Sherman et al., "Entecavir therapy for lamivudine-refractory chronic hepatitis B: Improved virologic, biochemical, and serology outcomes through 96 weeks," *Hepatology* 48 (2008), pp. 99–108.

189 In 1990, Dr. Joseph Murray of the Brigham and Women's Hospital in Boston, Massachusetts, with Dr. E. Donnall Thomas of the Fred Hutchinson Cancer Research Center, University of Washington, Seattle, shared the Nobel Prize for transplantation: Joseph E. Murray, Nobel Lecture, http://nobelprize.org/nobel_prizes/medicine/laureates/1990/murray-lecture.html.

190 The assessment of patients with advanced liver disease for transplantation and differences among different medical centers: Mohamad R. Al Sibae, Mitchell S. Cappell, "Accuracy of MELD scores in predicting mortality in decompensated cirrhosis from variceal bleed, hepatorenal syndrome, alcoholic hepatitis, or acute liver failure as well as mortality after non-transplant surgery or TIPS," *Digestive Diseases and Sciences* (Online First, September 1, 2010). Variation in waiting time: Jawad Ahmad et al., "Differences in access in liver transplantation: Disease severity, waiting time, and transplantation center volume," *Ann Intern Med* 146 (2007), pp. 707–713.

195 The comprehensive review of surrogate decision making: David Wendler, Annette Rid, "Systematic review: The effect on surrogates of making treatment decisions for others," *Ann Intern Med* 154 (2011), pp. 336–346.

195 Ethical principles involved in surrogate decision making: Ezekiel J. Emanuel, Linda L. Emanuel, "Proxy decision making for incompetent patients: An ethical and empirical analysis," *JAMA* 267 (1992), pp. 2067–2071; Alexia M. Torke, G. Caleb Alexander, John Lantos, "Substituted judgment: The limitations of autonomy in surrogate decision making," *JGIM* 23 (2008), pp. 1514–1517.

196 The research by Dr. Torke on the primary factor in physician decision making: Alexia M. Torke et al., "Physicians' views on the importance of patient preferences in surrogate decision-making," *Journal of the American Geriatrics Society* 58 (2010), pp. 533–538.

199 Further assessment of which principles surrogates rely on to make choices for incapacitated patients: Karen B. Hirschman, Jennifer M. Kapo, Jason H. T. Karlawish, "Why doesn't a family member of a person with advanced dementia use a substituted judgment when making a decision for that per-

son?" *American Journal of Geriatric Psychiatry* 14 (2006), pp. 659–667; Robert M. Arnold, John Kellum, "Moral justifications for surrogate decision making in the intensive care unit: Implications and limitations," *Critical Care Medicine* 31 (2003), pp. S347–S353.

199 Further analysis of how physicians weigh patient autonomy: Timothy E. Quill, Howard Brody, "Physician recommendations and patient autonomy: Finding a balance between physician power and patient choice," *Ann Intern Med* 125 (1996), pp. 763–769.

199 The potential limitation of the narrative approach is it does not provide a ready way to resolve disagreements about which treatments to select and which to forgo between surrogates and the doctors or among different surrogates. Furthermore, Dr. Torke points out there is no "objective scale for judging one family member's narrative is superior to another's." See Alexia M. Torke, G. Caleb Alexander, John Lantos, "Substituted judgment: The limitations of autonomy in surrogate decision making," *JGIM* 23 (2008), pp. 1514–1517.

203 Chris Klug's story: "Transplant survivor," www.chrisklug.com

205 The study from the United Kingdom on futility in the intensive care unit: Simon Atkinson et al., "Identification of futility in intensive care," *Lancet* 344 (1994), pp. 1203–1206. Different metrics to try to determine futility: "Consensus statement of the Society of Critical Care Medicine's Ethics Committee regarding futile and other possibly inadvisable treatment," *Critical Care Medicine* 5 (1997), pp. 887–891; European Society of Intensive Care Medicine Consensus Conference, "Predicting outcome in ICU patients," *Intensive Care Medicine* 20 (1994), pp. 390–397. The research from Paris on various patients considered for ICU admission and physician inability to accurately predict the outcome: Guillaume Thiery et al., "Outcome of cancer patients considered for intensive care unit admission: A hospital-wide prospective study," *JCO* 23 (2005), pp. 4406–4413. The study was conducted at Hôpital Saint-Louis in Paris, France, which has a large population of cancer patients. Among those predicted to die very soon, 26 percent were still alive 30 days later and 17 percent were alive 180 days later, clearly indicating that their prognosis was not so poor as to deny them care in the ICU. Similarly, cancer patients who were considered too well to benefit from ICU care had a death rate of 21 percent 30 days later, suggesting that they might have benefited from intensive treatment. Doctors' estimates were too optimistic and too pessimistic. A study of accuracy in predicting

outcomes for patients with terminal illness who are being discharged from the hospital to hospice: Nicholas A. Christakis, Elizabeth B. Lamont, "Extent and determinants of error in physicians' prognoses in terminally ill patients: Prospective cohort study," *Western Journal of Medicine* 172 (2000), pp. 310–313.

205 The mortality probability models: Stanley Lemeshow et al., "Mortality probability models (MPM II) based on an international cohort of intensive care unit patients," *JAMA* 270 (1993), pp. 2478–2486. The APACHE model: Task Force of the American College of Critical Care Medicine, Society of Critical Care Medicine, "Guidelines for intensive care unit admission, discharge, and triage," *Critical Care Medicine* 27 (1999), pp. 633–638.

206 Further debate about how to define futility: David B. Waisel, Robert D. Truog, "The cardiopulmonary resuscitation-not-indicated order: Futility revisited," *Ann Intern Med* 122 (1995), pp. 304–308; Richard S. Stein et al., "CPR-not-indicated and futility," *Ann Intern Med* 124 (1996), pp. 75–77; Stuart J. Youngner, "Who defines futility?" *JAMA* 260 (1988), pp. 2094–2095; Sofia Moratti, "The development of 'medical futility': Towards a procedural approach based on the role of the medical profession," *Journal of Medical Ethics* 35 (2009), pp. 369–372.

206 The essay by Dr. Veysman: Boris Veysman, "Shock me, tube me, line me," *Health Affairs* 29 (2010), pp. 324–326. Counterpoint essays from physicians with different perspectives: Victoria Sweet, "Thy will be done: Think your living will takes care of everything? Maybe not," *Health Affairs* 26 (2007), pp. 825–830; Victoria Sweet, "Code Pearl: In addition to full codes and DNRs, a physician calls for a new option that provides all life-prolonging treatments until death—and then a kind farewell," *Health Affairs* 27 (2008), pp. 216–220.

207 The proposal from the Clinical Guidelines Committee of the American College of Physicians to use QALYs in health care reform: Douglas K. Owens et al., "High-value, cost-conscious health care: Concepts for clinicians to evaluate the benefits, harms, and costs of medical interventions," *Ann Intern Med* 154 (2011), pp. 174–180. The caveats about setting a fixed cost to approve therapies: Michael K. Gusmano, Daniel Callahan, "Value for money: Use with care," *Ann Intern Med* 154 (2011), pp. 207–208. This includes discussion of NICE. The critique of QALYs: Paul Dolan, "Developing methods that really do value the 'Q' in the QALY," *Health Economics, Policy and Law* 3 (2008), pp. 69–77; Paul Dolan, "In defense of subjective well-being," *Health Economics, Policy and Law* 3 (2008), pp. 93–95; Paul

Dolan, Daniel Kahneman, "Interpretations of utility and their implications for the valuation of health," *Economic Journal* 118 (2008), pp. 215–234; Daniel Kahneman, "A different approach to health state valuation," special issue, *Value in Health* 12 (2009), pp. S16–S17. A defense of QALYs that we find unconvincing: Peter J. Neumann, "What next for QALYs?" *JAMA* (commentary) 305 (2011), pp. 1806–1807.

209 The use of narratives about a person's life to help inform surrogate choices: Mark G. Kuczewski, "Commentary: Narrative views of personal identity and substituted judgment in surrogate decision making," *Journal of Law, Medicine & Ethics* 27 (1999), pp. 32–36; Jeffrey Blustein, "Choosing for others as continuing a life story: The problem of personal identity revisited," *Journal of Law, Medicine & Ethics* 27 (1999), pp. 20–31.

Conclusion

212 The contention that the art of medicine is passé, to be replaced by industrialized medicine, with physicians following operating manuals and adhering strictly to standardized protocols: Stephen J. Swensen et al., "Cottage industry to postindustrial care: The revolution in health care delivery," *NEJM* 362 (2010), pp. E12(1)–E12(4); Robert H. Brook, "A physician = emotion + passion + science," *JAMA* 304 (2010), pp. 2528–2529; David Leonhardt, "Making health care better," *New York Times Magazine*, November 8, 2009. Also see unintended consequences of efficiency: Michael B. Edmond, "Taylorized medicine," *Ann Intern Med* 153 (2010), pp. 845–846.

212 Those who seek to standardize care base their argument largely on a study from the RAND Corporation claiming that on average, Americans receive only some 55 percent of "recommended care." The specific aspects of "recommended care" were designated by committees of "experts" convened by RAND. The RAND researchers then compared the expert recommendations with clinical practice in the United States, the latter assessed from retrospectively reviewing patient medical records. The RAND study has been criticized for relying on incomplete medical records and asserting that recommended care was essential to patient welfare when many of the recommendations were not proven to better health. Also recall how quickly recommendations of expert committees like the ones convened by RAND become outdated. See the original RAND study: Elizabeth A. McGlynn et al., "The quality of health care delivered to adults in the United States," *NEJM* 348 (2003), pp. 2635–2645. Flaws in the study: Correspondence to

Elizabeth A. McGlynn et al., "Quality of Health Care Delivered to Adults in the United States," *NEJM* 349 (2003), pp. 1866–1868. A subsequent study from Harvard researchers who implemented the care similar to that recommended by RAND in a real-world setting found no improvement in health outcomes of diabetes, asthma, and hypertension: Bruce E. Landon et al., "Improving the management of chronic disease at community health centers," *NEJM* 356 (2007), pp. 921–934. Commentary by Dr. Rodney Hayward on the failure of the RAND measures to succeed: Rodney A. Hayward, "Performance measurement in search of a path," *NEJM* 356 (2007), pp. 951–953. The report of expert recommendations becoming outdated: Kaveh G. Shojania et al., "How quickly do systematic reviews go out of date? A survival analysis," *Ann Intern Med* 147 (2007), pp. 224–233. Despite these cogent and long-standing criticisms of the RAND study published in 2003, the "fact" that Americans receive only some 55 percent of recommended care is widely quoted in presentations to the Congress and in the media: "What is health care quality and who decides?" Statement of Carolyn Clancy Before the Subcommittee on Health Care, March 18, 2009, Committee on Finance, U.S. Senate, http://www.ahrq.gov/news/test03 1809.htm; Donald Berwick et al., "Even good medical standards don't apply in all cases," Letters to the Editor, *Wall Street Journal*, April 15, 2009. Also see Jerome Groopman, Pamela Hartzband, "Sorting fact from fiction on health care," *Wall Street Journal*, August 31, 2009. Other recent studies showing failure of standardized quality measures to improve health outcomes, despite linkage of compliance with the measures to physician and hospital payment: Lauren H. Nicholas et al., "Hospital process compliance and surgical outcomes in Medicare beneficiaries," *Archives of Surgery* 145 (2010), pp. 999–1004; Charles D. Mabry, "Say it ain't so, Joe," *Archives of Surgery* 145 (2010), pp. 1004–1005. Also see Robert H. Brook, "The end of the quality improvement movement: Long live improving value," *JAMA* 304 (2010), pp. 1831–1832.

213 Studies on the use of so-called alternative and natural therapies in the United States: David Eisenberg et al., "Trends in alternative medicine use in the United States, 1990–1997: Results of a follow-up national survey," *JAMA* 280 (1998), pp. 1569–1575.

Selected Bibliography

Abramson, J., and J. M. Wright. "Are lipid-lowering guidelines evidence-based?" *Lancet* 369 (2007): 168–169.

Adams, John L., Ateev Mehrotra, J. William Thomas, and Elizabeth A. McGlynn. "Physician cost profiling: Reliability and risk of misclassification." *New England Journal of Medicine (NEJM)* 362 (2010): 1014–1021.

Action to Control Cardiovascular Risk in Diabetes Study Group. "Effects of intensive glucose lowering in Type 2 diabetes." *NEJM* 358 (2008): 2545–2559.

ADVANCE Collaborative Group. "Intensive blood glucose control and vascular outcomes in patients with Type 2 diabetes." *NEJM* 358 (2008): 2560–2572.

Agency for Healthcare Research and Quality. "Effective health care: Comparative effectiveness of therapies for clinically localized prostate cancer." *Executive Summary* (February 2008). http://www.effectivehealthcare.ahrq.gov/ehc/products/9/79/2008_0204ProstateCancerExecSum.pdf.

Ahmad, Jawad, et al. "Differences in access in liver transplantation: Disease severity, waiting time, and transplantation center volume." *Annals of Internal Medicine (Ann Intern Med)* 146 (2007): 707–713.

Al Sibae, Mohamad R., and Mitchell S. Cappell. "Accuracy of MELD scores in predicting mortality in decompensated cirrhosis from variceal bleed, hepatorenal syndrome, alcoholic hepatitis, or acute liver failure as well as mortality after nontransplant surgery or TIPS." *Digestive Diseases and Sciences* (Online First, September 1, 2010). DOI 10.1007/s10620-010-1390-3.

Andriole, Gerald L., et al. "Mortality results from a randomized prostate-cancer screening trial." *NEJM* 360 (2009): 1310–1319.

Ariely, Dan. *Predictably Irrational: The Hidden Forces That Shape Our Decisions.* New York: HarperCollins, 2008.

———. *The Upside of Irrationality: The Unexpected Benefits of Defying Logic at Work and at Home.* New York: HarperCollins, 2010.

Armstrong, Lance. *It's Not About the Bike: My Journey Back to Life,* Rei Rep ed. New York: Berkley Trade, 2001.

Atkinson, Simon, et al. "Identification of futility in intensive care." *Lancet* 344 (1994): 1203–1206.

Avorn, Jerry. *Powerful Medicines: The Benefits, Risks, and Costs of Prescription Drugs.* New York: Alfred A. Knopf, 2004.

Ball, W. W. Rouse. *A Short Account of the History of Mathematics,* 4th ed. Mineola, NY: Dover Publications, 2010.

Barry, Michael J. "Screening for prostate cancer: The controversy that refuses to die." *NEJM* 360 (2009): 1351–1354.

Beasley, B. Nhi, Ellis F. Unger, and Robert Temple. "Anticoagulant options: Why the FDA approved a higher but not a lower dose of dabigatran." *NEJM* (Online First, April 13, 2011).

Berwick, Donald. "My right knee." *Ann Intern Med* 142 (2005): 121–125.

———. "What 'patient-centered' should mean: Confessions of an extremist." *Health Affairs—Web Exclusive* 28, no. 4 (2009): W555–W565.

Berwick, Donald, et al. "Even good medical standards don't apply in all cases." Letters to the Editor. *Wall Street Journal,* April 15, 2009.

Bhattacharyya, Timothy, et al. "Measuring the report card: The validity of pay-for-performance metrics in orthopedic surgery." *Health Affairs* 28 (2009): 526–532.

Bill-Axelson, Anna, et al. "Radical prostatectomy versus watchful waiting in early prostate cancer." *NEJM* 352 (2005): 1977–1984.

Blumberg, Baruch S. "The Nobel Prize in Physiology or Medicine 1976." Baruch S. Blumberg, Autobiography. http://nobelprize.org/nobel_prizes/medicine/laureates/1976/blumberg-autobio.html.

Blustein, Jeffrey. "Choosing for others as continuing a life story: The problem of personal identity revisited." *Journal of Law, Medicine & Ethics* 27 (1999): 20–31.

Boyd, Norman F., et al. "Whose utilities for decision analysis?" *Medical Decision Making* 10 (1990): 58–67.

Brent, Gregory A. "Graves' disease." *NEJM* 358 (2008): 2594–2605.

Broedl, Uli C., Hans-Christian Geiss, and Klaus G. Parhofer. "Comparison of current guidelines for primary prevention of coronary heart disease." *Journal of General Internal Medicine* (*JGIM*) 18 (2003): 190–195.

Brook, Robert H. "A physician = emotion + passion + science." *Journal of the American Medical Association* (*JAMA*) 304 (2010): 2528–2529.

———. "The end of the quality improvement movement: Long live improving value." *JAMA* 304 (2010): 1831–1832.

Bruni, Frank. "Death takes a rain check: How many blueberries a day does it take to keep the grim reaper away? An 87-year-old billionaire's quest to live forever— or at least to 125." *New York Times Magazine,* March 6, 2011.

Chapman, Gretchen B., et al. "Prostate cancer patients' utilities for health states: How it looks depends on where you stand." *Medical Decision Making* 18 (1998): 278–286.

Chapman, Gretchen B. "The psychology of medical decision making." In D. J. Koehler and N. Harvey (eds.). *Blackwell Handbook of Judgment and Decision Making.* Oxford, UK: Blackwell Publishing, 2004, pp. 585–603.

Cheung, Bernard M. Y., and Karen S. L. Lam. "Is intensive LDL-cholesterol lowering beneficial and safe?" *Lancet* 376 (2010): 1622–1623.

Chlebowski, Rowan T., et al. "Estrogen plus progestin and breast cancer incidence and mortality in postmenopausal women." *JAMA* 304 (2010): 1684–1692.

Chobanian, Avram V., et al. "The Seventh Report of the Joint National Committee on Prevention, Detection, Evaluation, and Treatment of High Blood Pressure: The JNC 7 Report." *JAMA* 289 (2003): 2560–2572.

Christakis, Nicholas A., and Elizabeth B. Lamont. "Extent and determinants of error in physicians' prognoses in terminally ill patients: Prospective cohort study." *Western Journal of Medicine* 172 (2000): 310–313.

Chua, Hannah Faye, et al. "Decision-related loss: Regret and disappointment." *NeuroImage* 47 (2009): 2031–2040.

Clancy, Carolyn. "What is health care quality and who decides?" Statement of Carolyn Clancy Before the Subcommittee on Health Care, March 18, 2009. Committee on Finance, U.S. Senate. http://www.ahrq.gov/news/test031809.htm.

Collins, Francis S. *The Language of Life: DNA and the Revolution in Personalized Medicine.* New York: HarperCollins, 2010.

Collins, Gail. "Medicine on the move." *New York Times* (op-ed), April 7, 2011.

Colwell, Janet. "Should doctors worry about online ratings?" *ACP Internist* 30 (2010): 1, 16.

Connolly, Stuart J., et al. "Dabigatran versus warfarin in patients with atrial fibrillation." *NEJM* 361 (2009): 1139–1151.

Connolly, Terry, et al. "Regret and responsibility in the evaluation of decision outcomes." *Organizational Behavior and Human Decision Processes* 70 (1997): 73–85.

Connolly, Terry, and Marcel Zeelenberg. "Regret in decision making." *Current Directions in Psychological Science* 11 (2002): 212–216.

Connolly, Terry, and Jochen Reb. "Regret in cancer-related decisions." *Health Psychology* 24 (2005): S29–S34.

"Consensus statement of the Society of Critical Care Medicine's Ethics Committee regarding futile and other possibly inadvisable treatment." *Critical Care Medicine* 5 (1997): 887–891.

Conway, Patrick, and Carolyn Clancy. "Comparative-effectiveness research: Implications of the federal coordinating council's report." *NEJM* 361 (2009): 328–330.

Cousins, Norman. *Anatomy of an Illness as Perceived by the Patient.* New York: Bantam Doubleday Dell, 1981.

Couzin, Jennifer. "Cholesterol veers off script." *Science* 322 (2008): 220–223.

Couzin-Frankel, Jennifer. "U.S. panel favors wider use of preventive drug treatment." *Science* 327 (2010): 130–131.

Damberg, Cheryl L., et al. "Taking stock of pay-for-performance: A candid assessment from the front lines." *Health Affairs* 28 (2009): 517–525.

Damschroder, Laura J., Brian J. Zikmund-Fisher, and Peter A. Ubel. "Considering adaptation in preference elicitations." *Health Psychology* 27 (2008): 394–399.

Degner, Lesley F., et al. "Information needs and decisional preferences in women with breast cancer." *JAMA* 277 (1997): 1485–1492.

Devereaux, P. J., et al. "Differences between perspectives of physicians and patients on anticoagulation in patients with atrial fibrillation: Observational study." *British Medical Journal* 323 (2001): 1218–1222.

DiBonaventura, Marco daCosta, and Gretchen Chapman. "Do decision biases predict bad decisions? Omission bias, naturalness bias, and influenza vaccination." *Medical Decision Making* 28 (2008): 532–539.

Ditto, Peter H., et al. "Context changes choices: A prospective study of the effects of hospitalization on life-sustaining treatment preferences." *Medical Decision Making* 26 (2006): 313–322.

Ditto, Peter H., and Nikki A. Hawkins. "Advance directives and cancer decision making near the end of life." *Health Psychology* 24, Suppl. 4 (2005): S63–S70.

Dluhy, Robert G., and Graham T. McMahon. "Intensive glycemic control in the ACCORD and ADVANCE trials." *NEJM* 358 (2008): 2630–2633.

Dolan, Paul. "Developing methods that really do value the 'Q' in the QALY." *Health Economics, Policy and Law* 3 (2008): 69–77.

Dolan, Paul, and Daniel Kahneman. "Interpretations of utility and their implications for the valuation of health." *Economic Journal* 118 (2008): pp. 215–234.

Domanski, Michael J. "Primary prevention of coronary artery disease." *NEJM* 357 (2007): 1543–1545.

Domchek, Susan M., et al. "Association of risk-reducing surgery in BRCA1 or BRCA2 mutation carriers with cancer risk and mortality." *JAMA* 304 (2010): 967–975.

Edmond, Michael B. "Taylorized medicine." *Ann Intern Med* 153 (2010): 845–846.

Eisenberg, David, et al. "Trends in alternative medicine use in the United States, 1990–1997: Results of a follow-up national survey." *JAMA* 280 (1998): 1569–1575.

Elstein, Arthur S., et al. "Agreement between prostate cancer patients and their clinicians about utilities and attribute importance." *Health Expectations* 7 (2004): 115–125.

Elstein, Arthur S., Gretchen B. Chapman, and Sara J. Knight. "Patients' values and clinical substituted judgments: The case of localized prostate cancer." *Health Psychology* 24 (2005): S85–S92.

Emanuel, Ezekiel J., and Linda L. Emanuel. "Proxy decision making for incompetent patients: An ethical and empirical analysis." *JAMA* 267 (1992): 2067–2071.

Epstein, Ronald M., and Ellen Peters. "Beyond information: Exploring patients' preferences." *JAMA* 302 (2009): 195–197.

European Society of Intensive Care Medicine Consensus Conference. "Predicting outcome in ICU patients." *Intensive Care Medicine* 20 (1994): 390–397.

Favus, Murray J. "Bisphosphonates for osteoporosis." *NEJM* 363 (2010): 2027–2035.

Fonarow, Gregg C., et al. "Association between performance measures and clinical outcomes for patients hospitalized with heart failure." *JAMA* 297 (2007): 61–70.

Ford, Ian, et al. "Long-term follow-up of the West of Scotland Coronary Prevention Study." *NEJM* 357 (2007): 1477–1486.

Fraenkel, Liana, and Terri R. Fried. "Individualized medical decision making." *Archives of Internal Medicine* 170 (2010): 66–569.

Fried, Terri R., et al. "Prospective study of health status preferences and changes in preferences over time in older adults." *Archives of Internal Medicine* 166 (2006): 890–895.

———. "Inconsistency over time in the preferences of older persons with advanced illness for life-sustaining treatment." *Journal of the American Geriatrics Society* 55 (2007): 1007–1014.

Fried, Terri R., and John R. O'Leary. "Using the experience of bereaved caregivers to inform patient- and caregiver-centered advance care planning." *JGIM* 23 (2008): 1602–1607.

Frosch, Dominick L., et al. "Creating demand for prescription drugs: A content analysis of television direct-to-consumer advertising." *Annals of Family Medicine* 5 (2007): 6–13.

Gage, Brian F. "Can we rely on RE-LY?" *NEJM* 361 (2009): 1200–1202.

Gardner, Howard. *Changing Minds: The Art and Science of Changing Our Own and Other People's Minds.* Boston: Harvard Business School Press, 2006.

Gilbert, Daniel. *Stumbling on Happiness.* New York: Vintage Books, 2007.

Gilbert, Daniel, and Timothy D. Wilson. "Prospection: Experiencing the future." *Science* 317 (2007): 1351–1354.

Gilbert, Daniel T., et al. "The surprising power of neighborly advice." *Science* 323 (2009): 1617–1619.

Gillick, Muriel R. "Reversing the code status of advance directives?" *NEJM* 362 (2010): 1239–1240.

Go, Alan S., et al. "Prevalence of diagnosed atrial fibrillation in adults: National implications for rhythm management and stroke prevention: The Anticoagulation and Risk Factors in Atrial Fibrillation (ATRIA) Study." *JAMA* 285 (2001): 2370–2375.

Goetz, Thomas. *The Decision Tree: Taking Control of Your Health in the New Era of Personalized Medicine.* New York: Rodale Books, 2010.

Golub, Sarit A., and Daniel T. Gilbert. "Anticipating one's troubles: The costs and benefits of negative expectations." *Emotion* 9 (2009): 277–281.

Gould, Stephen Jay. "The median isn't the message." CancerGuide. http://cancerguide.org/median_not_msg.html.

Gribben, John G. "How I treat CLL up front." *Blood* 115 (2010): 187–197.

Groopman, Jerome. "A knife in the back: Is surgery the best approach to chronic back pain?" *New Yorker,* April 8, 2002.

———. *The Anatomy of Hope: How People Prevail in the Face of Illness.* New York: Random House, 2004.

———. *How Doctors Think.* New York: Houghton Mifflin, 2007.

———. "Health care: Who knows 'best'?" *New York Review of Books* 57 (2010): 12–15.

Groopman, Jerome, and Pamela Hartzband. "Sorting fact from fiction on health care." *Wall Street Journal,* August 31, 2009.

Gusmano, Michael K., and Daniel Callahan. "Value for money: Use with care." *Ann Intern Med* 154 (2011): 207–208. This includes discussion of NICE.

Hadler, Nortin M. *Worried Sick: A Prescription for Health in an Overtreated America.* Chapel Hill: University of North Carolina Press, 2008.

Halpern, Jodi, and Robert M. Arnold. "Affective forecasting: An unrecognized challenge in making serious health decisions." *JGIM* 23 (2008): 1708–1712.

Harrington, Anne. *The Cure Within: A History of Mind-Body Medicine.* New York: W. W. Norton & Co., 2008.

Hart, Robert G., Lesly A. Pearce, and Maria I. Aguilar. "Meta-analysis: Antithrombotic therapy to prevent stroke in patients who have nonvalvular atrial fibrillation." *Ann Intern Med* 146 (2007): 857–867.

Hartzband, Pamela, and Jerome Groopman. "Keeping the patient in the equation: Humanism and health care reform." *NEJM* 361 (2009): 554–555.

Hayward, Rodney A., Timothy P. Hofer, and Sandeep Vijan. "Narrative review: Lack of evidence for recommended low-density lipoprotein treatment targets: A solvable problem." *Ann Intern Med* 145 (2006): 520–530.

Hayward, Rodney A. "Performance measurement in search of a path." *NEJM* 356 (2007): 951–953.

Herrinton, Lisa J., et al. "Efficacy of prophylactic mastectomy in women with unilateral breast cancer: A cancer research network project." *Journal of Clinical Oncology (JCO)* 23 (2005): 4275–4286.

Hill, Catherine L., et al. "Frequency of specific cancer types in dermatomyositis and polymyositis: A population-based study." *Lancet* 357 (2001): 96–100.

Horning, Sandra J. "Risk, cure and complications in advanced Hodgkin disease." *Hematology* 1 (2007): 197–203.

Hu, Jim C., et al. "Comparative effectiveness of minimally invasive vs. open radical prostatectomy." *JAMA* 302 (2009): 1557–1564.

Hylek, Elaine M., et al. "Effect of intensity of oral anticoagulation on stroke severity and mortality in atrial fibrillation." *NEJM* 349 (2003): 1019–1026.

Institute of Medicine (National Academy of Sciences). *Crossing the Quality Chasm: A New Health System for the 21st Century*. Washington, DC: National Academy Press, 2001. http://www.nap.edu/books/0309072808/html.

Inzucchi, Silvio E., and Mark D. Siegel. "Glucose control in the ICU: How tight is too tight?" *NEJM* 360 (2009): 1346–1349.

Ioannidis, John P. A. "Contradicted and initially stronger effects in highly cited clinical research." *JAMA* 294 (2005): 218–228.

Joy, Tisha R., and Robert A. Hegele. "Narrative review: Statin-related myopathy." *Ann Intern Med* 150 (2009): 858–868.

Jungheim, Emily S., and Graham A. Colditz. "Short-term use of unopposed estrogen: A balance of inferred risks and benefits." *JAMA* 305 (2011): 1354–1355.

Kahneman, Daniel. "A different approach to health state valuation." Special issue, *Value in Health* 12 (2009): S16–S17.

Kahneman, Daniel, et al. "When more pain is preferred to less: Adding a better end." *Psychological Science* 4 (1993): 401–405.

———. "Would you be happier if you were richer? A focusing illusion." *Science* 312 (2006): 1908–1910.

Kahneman, Daniel, and Amos Tversky. "The psychology of preferences." *Scientific American* 246 (1982): 160–173.

Kahneman, Daniel, Jack L. Knetsch, and Richard H. Thaler. "The endowment effect, loss aversion, and status quo bias." *Journal of Economic Perspectives* 5 (1991): 193–206.

Keirns, Carla C., and Susan Dorr Goold. "Patient-centered care and preference-sensitive decision making." *JAMA* 302 (2009): 1085–1086.

Kelley, Amy S., and Diane E. Meier. "Palliative care: A shifting paradigm." *NEJM* 363 (2010): 781–782.

Knight, Sara J., et al. "Pilot study of a utilities-based treatment decision intervention for prostate cancer patients." *Clinical Prostate Cancer* 1 (September 2002): 105–114.

Kuczewski, Mark G. "Commentary: Narrative views of personal identity and substituted judgment in surrogate decision making." *Journal of Law, Medicine & Ethics* 27 (1999): 32–36.

Küppers, Ralf. "The biology of Hodgkin's lymphoma." *Nature Reviews Cancer* 9 (2009): 15–27.

Lacey, Heather P., et al. "Are they really that happy? Exploring scale recalibration in estimates of well-being." *Health Psychology* 27 (2008): 669–675.

LaCroix, Andrea Z., et al. "Health outcomes after stopping conjugated equine estrogens among postmenopausal women with prior hysterectomy: A randomized controlled trial." *JAMA* 305 (2011): 1305–1314.

Landon, Bruce E., et al. "Improving the management of chronic disease at community health centers." *NEJM* 356 (2007): 921–934.

Landro, Laura. "New efforts to simplify end-of-life care wishes." *Wall Street Journal,* March 15, 2011.

LeBlanc, Annie, David A. Kenny, Annette M. O'Connor, and France Legare. "Decisional conflict in patients and their physicians: A dyadic approach to shared decision making." *Medical Decision Making* 29 (2009): 61–68.

Legare, France, et al. "The effect of decision aids on the agreement between women's and physicians' decisional conflict about hormone replacement therapy." *Patient Education and Counseling* 50 (2003): 211–221.

Lemeshow, Stanley, et al. "Mortality probability models (MPM II) based on an international cohort of intensive care unit patients." *JAMA* 270 (1993): 2478–2486.

Leonhardt, David. "Making health care better." *New York Times Magazine,* November 8, 2009.

Lerman, Caryn, et al. "Prophylactic surgery decisions and surveillance practices one year following BRCA1/2 testing." *Preventive Medicine* 31 (2000): 75–80.

Levy, Daniel, and Susan Brink. *A Change of Heart: How the People of Framingham, Massachusetts, Helped Unravel the Mysteries of Cardiovascular Disease.* New York: Alfred A. Knopf, 2005.

Liang, Bryan A., and Timothy Mackey. "Direct-to-consumer advertising with interactive internet media: Global regulation and public health issues." *JAMA* 305 (2011): 824–825.

Lichtenstein, Sarah, and Paul Slovic. "The construction of preference: An overview." In Lichtenstein and Slovic (eds.). *The Construction of Preference.* New York: Cambridge University Press, 2006.

Litwin, Mark S., et al. "Quality of life after surgery, external beam irradiation, or brachytherapy for early-stage prostate cancer." *Cancer* 109 (2007): 2239–2247.

Llewellyn-Thomas, Hilary A., et al. "Studying patients' preferences in health care decision making." *Canadian Medical Association Journal (CMAJ)* 147 (1992): 859–864.

Lloyd-Jones, Donald M., et al. "Lifetime risk for development of atrial fibrillation: The Framingham Heart Study." *Circulation* 110 (2004): 1042–1046.

Loewenstein, George. "Hot-cold empathy gaps and medical decision making." *Health Psychology* 24 (2005): S49–S56.

Loewenstein, George, and David Schkade. "Wouldn't it be nice? Predicting future feelings." In D. Kahneman, E. Diener, and N. Schwarz (eds.). *Well-Being: The Foundation of Hedonic Psychology.* New York: Russell Sage Foundation, 1998, pp. 85–105.

Luce, Mary Frances. "Decision making as coping." *Health Psychology* 24 (2005): S23–S28.

Mabry, Charles D. "Say it ain't so, Joe." *Archives of Surgery* 145 (2010): 1004–1005.

MacTutor History of Mathematics Archive. "Daniel Bernoulli." Index of biographies. http://www-history.mcs.st-and.ac.uk/Biographies/Bernoulli_Daniel.html.

Mancia, Giuseppe, et al. "2007 guidelines for the management of arterial hypertension: The Task Force for the Management of Arterial Hypertension of the European Society of Hypertension (ESH) and of the European Society of Cardiology (ESC)." *Journal of Hypertension* 25 (2007): 1105–1187.

Man-Son-Hing, Malcolm, et al. "The effect of qualitative vs. quantitative presentation of probability estimates on patient decision-making: A randomized trial." *Health Expectations* 5 (2002): 246–255.

Marder, Jenny. "A user's guide to cancer treatment." *Science* 326 (2009): 1184.

Marks, Lawrence B., et al. "One to three versus four or more positive nodes and postmastectomy radiotherapy: Time to end the debate." *JCO* 26 (2008): 2075–2077.

McAlister, Finlay A. "Applying evidence to patient care: From black and white to shades of grey." *Ann Intern Med* 138 (2003): 938–939.

McAlister, Finlay A., et al. "When should hypertension be treated? The different perspectives of Canadian family physicians and patients." *CMAJ* 163 (2000): 403–408.

———. "Users' guides to the medical literature: Integrating research evidence with the care of the individual patient." *JAMA* 283 (2000): 2829–2836.

———. "How evidence-based are the recommendations in evidence-based guidelines?" *PLoS Medicine* 4 (2007): 1325–1332.

McGlynn, Elizabeth A., et al., "The quality of health care delivered to adults in the United States." *NEJM* 348 (2003): 2635–2645.

McNeil, Barbara J., Stephen G. Pauker, Harold C. Sox, and Amos Tversky. "On the elicitation of preferences for alternative therapies." *NEJM* 306 (1982): 1259–1269.

McNutt, Robert A. "Shared medical decision making: Problems, process, progress." *JAMA* 292 (2002): 2516–2518.

Meier, Diane E., and Larry Beresford. "POLST offers next stage in honoring patient preferences." *Journal of Palliative Medicine* 12 (2009): 291–295.

Metcalfe, Kelly A., et al. "International variation in rates of uptake of preventive options in BRCA1 and BRCA2 mutation carriers." *International Journal of Cancer* 122 (2008): 2017–2022.

Miller, Nancy Houston. "Compliance with treatment regimens in chronic asymptomatic diseases." *American Journal of Medicine* 102 (1997): 43–49.

Montserrat, Emili, et al. "How I treat refractory CLL." *Blood* 107 (2006): 1276–1283.

Morewedge, Carey K., Daniel T. Gilbert, and Timothy D. Wilson. "The least likely of times: How remembering the past biases forecasts of the future." *Psychological Science* 16 (2005): 626–630.

Moseley, J. Bruce, et al. "A controlled trial of arthroscopic surgery for osteoarthritis of the knee." *NEJM* 347 (2002): 81–88.

Murray, Joseph E. Nobel Lecture. http://nobelprize.org/nobel_prizes/medicine/laureates/1990/murray-lecture.html.

Naccarelli, Gerald V., et al. "Increasing prevalence of atrial fibrillation and flutter in the United States." *American Journal of Cardiology* 104 (2009): 1534–1539.

Naglie, Gary, et al. "Primer on medical decision analysis: Estimating probabilities and utilities." *Medical Decision Making* 136 (1997): 136–141.

National Community Pharmacists Association. "Enhancing prescription medicine adherence: A national action plan." Rockville, MD: National Council on Patient Information and Education, August 2007, p. 7.

Neumann, John von, and Oskar Morgenstern. *Theory of Games and Economic Behavior*, 2nd ed. Princeton, NJ: Princeton University Press, 1947.

NICE-SUGAR Study Investigators. "Intensive versus conventional glucose control in critically ill patients." *NEJM* 360 (2009): 1283–1297.

Nicholas, Lauren H., et al. "Hospital process compliance and surgical outcomes in Medicare beneficiaries." *Archives of Surgery* 145 (2010): 999–1004.

Ofri, Danielle. "Quality measures and the individual physician." *NEJM* 363 (2010): 606–607.

Ong, Michael K., et al. "Looking forward, looking back: Assessing variations in hospital resource use and outcomes for elderly patients with heart failure." *Circulation Cardiovascular Quality and Outcomes* 2 (2009): 548–557.

Osterberg, Lars, and Terrence Blaschke. "Adherence to medication." *NEJM* 353 (2005): 487–497.

Owens, Douglas K., et al. "High-value, cost-conscious health care: Concepts for clinicians to evaluate the benefits, harms, and costs of medical interventions." *Ann Intern Med* 154 (2011): 174–180.

Parker-Pope, Tara. "Estrogen lowers breast cancer and heart attack risk in some." *New York Times* (Well), April 6, 2011.

Pauker, Stephen G., and Jerome P. Kassirer. "Decision analysis." *NEJM* 316 (1987): 250–258.

Paulos, John Allen. "Metric mania." *New York Times Magazine*, May 16, 2010.

Payne, David K., et al. "Women's regrets after bilateral prophylactic mastectomy." *Annals of Surgical Oncology* 7 (2000): 150–154.

Penson, David F., et al. "5-year urinary and sexual outcomes after radical prostatectomy: Results from the prostate cancer outcomes study." *Journal of Urology* 173 (2005): 1701–1705.

Perrillo, Robert P., and Andrew L. Mason. "Hepatitis B and liver transplantation: Problems and promises." *NEJM* 329 (1993): 1885–1887.

Pinker, Steven. "My genome, my self." *New York Times Magazine*, January 11, 2009.

Puchalski, Christina M., et al. "Patients who want their family and physician to make resuscitation decisions for them: Observations from SUPPORT and HELP." *Journal of the American Geriatrics Society* 48 (2000): S84–S90.

Qaseem, Amir, et al., "The development of clinical practice guidelines and guidance statements of the American College of Physicians: Summary of methods." *Ann Intern Med* 153 (2010): 194–199.

Quanstrum, Kerianne H., and Rodney A. Hayward. "Lessons from the mammography wars." *NEJM* 363 (2010): 1076–1079.

Quill, Timothy E., and Howard Brody. "Physician recommendations and patient autonomy: Finding a balance between physician power and patient choice." *Ann Intern Med* 125 (1996): 763–769.

Quill, Timothy E. "Initiating end-of-life discussions with seriously ill patients: Addressing the 'elephant in the room.'" *JAMA* 284 (2000): 2502–2507.

Rabin, Roni Caryn. "Perceptions: Doctors, patients and a clash of priorities." *New York Times*, February 9, 2010.

Ragaz, Joseph, et al. "Locoregional radiation therapy in patients with high-risk breast cancer receiving adjuvant chemotherapy: 20-year results of the British Columbia randomized trial." *Journal of the National Cancer Institute* 97 (2005): 116–126.

Raymont, Vanessa, et al. "Prevalence of mental incapacity in medical inpatients and associated risk factors: Cross-sectional study." *Lancet* 364 (2004): 1421–1427.

Redelmeier, Donald A., Paul Rozin, and Daniel Kahneman. "Understanding patients' decisions: Cognitive and emotional perspectives." *JAMA* 270 (1993): 72–76.

Resnic, Frederick S., and Frederick G. P. Welt. "The public health hazards of risk avoidance associated with public reporting of risk-adjusted outcomes in coronary intervention." *Journal of the American College of Cardiology* 53 (2009): 825–830.

Roter, Debra, and Judith A. Hall. *Doctors Talking with Patients/Patients Talking with Doctors.* Westport, CT: Praeger Publishing, 2006.

Sawyer, Susan M., and H. John Fardy. "Bridging the gap between doctors' and patients' expectations of asthma management." *Journal of Asthma* 40 (2003): 131–138.

Schkade, David A., and Daniel Kahneman. "Does living in California make people happy? A focusing illusion in judgments of life satisfaction." *Psychological Science* 9 (1998): 340–346.

Schneider, Carl E. *The Practice of Autonomy: Patients, Doctors, and Medical Decisions.* New York: Oxford University Press, 1998.

Schroder, Fritz H., et al. "Screening and prostate-cancer mortality in a randomized European study." *NEJM* 360 (2009): 1320–1328.

Schwartz, Alan, and George Bergus. *Medical Decision Making: A Physician's Guide.* Cambridge, UK: Cambridge University Press, 2008.

Schwartz, Barry. "Tyranny of Choice." *Scientific American* 290 (2004): 70–75.

———. *The Paradox of Choice.* New York: Harper Perennial, 2005.

Schwartz, Barry, and Jim Weinstein. "Partnership: Doctor and patient." *Spine* 30 (2005): 269–271.

Schwartz, Lisa M., et al. "Using a drug facts box to communicate drug benefits and harms: Two randomized trials." *Ann Intern Med* 150 (2009): 516–527.

Schwartz, Marc D., et al. "Bilateral prophylactic oophorectomy and ovarian cancer screening following BRCA1/BRCA2 mutation testing. *JCO* 21 (2003): 4034–4041.

———. "Impact of BRCA1/BRCA2 counseling and testing on newly diagnosed breast cancer patients." *JCO* 22 (2004): 1823–1829.

———. "Utilization of BRCA1/BRCA2 mutation testing in newly diagnosed breast cancer patients." *Cancer Epidemiology, Biomarkers & Prevention* 14 (2005): 1003–1007.

———. "Decision making and decision support for hereditary breast-ovarian cancer susceptibility." *Health Psychology* (2005): S78–S84.

Sears, Sharon R., Annette L. Stanton, and Sharon Daoff-Burg. "The yellow brick road and the emerald city: Benefit finding, positive reappraisal coping, and post-traumatic growth in women with early-stage breast cancer." *Health Psychology* 22 (2003): 487–497.

Sepucha, Karen R., et al. "Developing instruments to measure the quality of decisions: Early results for a set of symptom-driven decisions." *Patient Education and Counseling* 73 (2008): 504–510.

Sevdalis, Nick, and Nigel Harvey. "Predicting preferences: A neglected aspect of shared decision-making." *Health Expectations* 9 (2006): 245–251.

Sewitch, Maida J., et al. "Measuring differences between patients' and physicians' health perceptions: The patient-physician discordance scale." *Journal of Behavioral Medicine* 26 (2003): 245–264.

Shekelle, Paul G., et al. "Validity of the Agency for Healthcare Research and Quality clinical practice guidelines: How quickly do guidelines become outdated?" *JAMA* 286 (2001): 1461–1467.

Sherman, Morris, et al. "Entecavir therapy for lamivudine-refractory chronic hepatitis B: Improved virologic, biochemical, and serology outcomes through 96 weeks." *Hepatology* 48 (2008): 99–108.

Shojania, Kaveh G., et al. "How quickly do systematic reviews go out of date? A survival analysis." *Ann Intern Med* 147 (2007): 224–233.

Siris, Ethel S., et al. "Adherence to bisphosphonate therapy, vitamin D and calcium supplements and fracture rates in osteoporotic women: Relationship to vertebral and nonvertebral fractures from 2 US claims databases." *Mayo Clinic Proceedings* 81 (2006): 1013–1022.

Slater, Jerry D., et al. "Proton therapy for prostate cancer: The initial Loma Linda University experience." *International Journal of Radiation Oncology, Biology, Physics* 59 (2004): 348–352.

Slovic, Paul. "Perception of risk." *Science* 236 (1987): 280–285.

Slovic, Paul, et al. "Affect, risk, and decision making." *Health Psychology* 24 (2005): S35–S40.

Smith, Dylan M., et al. "Misremembering colostomies? Former patients give lower utility ratings than do current patients." *Health Psychology* 25 (2006): 688–695.

Smolen, Josef S. "Therapy of systemic lupus erythematosus: A look into the future." *Arthritis Research* 4, Suppl. 3 (2002): S25–S30.

Sniderman, Allan D., and Curt D. Furberg. "Why guideline-making requires reform." *JAMA* 301 (2009): 429–431.

Spiro, Howard. *The Power of Hope: A Doctor's Perspective.* New Haven, CT: Yale University Press, 1998.

Spoorenberg, A., et al. "Measuring disease activity in ankylosing spondylitis: Patient and physician have different perspectives." *Rheumatology* (Oxford) 44 (2005): 789–795.

Sudore, Rebecca L., and Terri R. Fried. "Redefining the 'planning' in advance care planning: Preparing for end-of-life decision making." *Ann Intern Med* 153 (2010): 256–261.

Sudore, Rebecca L., Dean Schillinger, Sara J. Knight, and Terri R. Fried. "Uncertainty about advance care planning treatment preferences among diverse older adults." *Journal of Health Communication* 15, Suppl. 2 (2010): 159–171.

SUPPORT Principal Investigators. "A controlled trial to improve care for seriously ill hospitalized patients: The study to understand prognoses and preferences for outcomes and risks of treatments (SUPPORT)." *JAMA* 274 (1995): 1591–1598.

Sweet, Victoria. "Thy will be done: Think your living will takes care of everything? Maybe not." *Health Affairs* 26 (2007): 825–830.

Swensen, Stephen J., et al. "Cottage industry to postindustrial care: The revolution in health care delivery." *NEJM* 362 (2010): E12(1)–E12(4).

Task Force of the American College of Critical Care Medicine, Society of Critical Care Medicine. "Guidelines for intensive care unit admission, discharge, and triage." *Critical Care Medicine* 27 (1999): 633–638.

Temel, Jennifer S., et al. "Early palliative care for patients with metastatic non-small-cell lung cancer." *NEJM* 363 (2010): 733–742.

Thaler, Richard H., and Cass R. Sunstein. *Nudge: Improving Decisions About Health, Wealth, and Happiness.* New York: Penguin Books, 2009.

Thiery, Guillaume, et al. "Outcome of cancer patients considered for intensive care unit admission: A hospital-wide prospective study." *JCO* 23 (2005): 4406–4413.

"Third report of the National Cholesterol Education Program (NCEP) expert panel on detection, evaluation, and treatment of high blood cholesterol in adults (Adult Treatment Panel III)." *Circulation* 106 (2002): 3143–3421.

Thomas, E. Donnall. Autobiography. Nobelprize.org. http://nobelprize.org/ nobel_prizes/medicine/laureates/1990/thomas-autobio.html.

Tinetti, Mary E. "Potential pitfalls of disease-specific guidelines for patients with multiple conditions." *NEJM* 351 (2004): 2870–2874.

Torke, Alexia M., G. Caleb Alexander, and John Lantos. "Substituted judgment: The limitations of autonomy in surrogate decision making." *JGIM* 23 (2008): 1514–1517.

Torke, Alexia M., et al. "Physicians' views on the importance of patient preferences in surrogate decision-making." *Journal of the American Geriatrics Society* 58 (2010): 533–538.

Torring, Ove, et al. "Graves' hyperthyroidism: Treatment with antithyroid drugs, surgery, or radioiodine—a prospective, randomized study: Thyroid Study Group." *Journal of Clinical Endocrinology & Metabolism* 81 (1996): 2986–2993.

Tu, Ha T., and Johanna R. Lauer. "Word of mouth and physician referrals still drive health care provider choice." *HSC Research Brief* (Center for Studying Health System Change, Washington, DC) 9 (December 2008).

Tversky, Amos, and Daniel Kahneman. "The framing of decisions and the psychology of choice." *Science* 211 (1981): 453–458.

Tversky, Amos, and Eldar Shafir. "Choice under conflict: The dynamics of deferred decision." *Psychological Science* 3 (1992): 358–361.

Ubel, Peter A., et al. "What is perfect health to an 85-year-old? Evidence for scale recalibration in subjective health ratings." *Medical Care* 43 (2005): 1054–1057.

———. "Misimaging the unimaginable: The disability paradox in health care decision making." *Health Psychology* 24 (2005): S57–S62.

United States Department of Health and Human Services/National Heart, Lung, and Blood Institute. "Health information for the public." http://www .nhlbi.nih.gov/health.

Venkitaraman, Ashok R. "Cancer susceptibility and the functions of BRCA1 and BRCA2." *Cell* 108 (2002): 171–182.

Verghese, Abraham. "Treat the patient, not the CT scan." *New York Times*, February 27, 2011.

Veysman, Boris. "Shock me, tube me, line me." *Health Affairs* 29 (2010): 324–326.

Wartofsky, Leonard, et al. "Differences and similarities in the diagnosis and treatment of Graves' disease in Europe, Japan, and the United States." *Thyroid* 1 (1991): 129–135.

Weinstein, James N., Kate Clay, and Tamara S. Morgan. "Informed patient choice: Patient-centered valuing of surgical risks and benefits." *Health Affairs* 26 (2007): 726–730.

Welch, H. Gilbert. *Overdiagnosed: Making People Sick in the Pursuit of Health.* Boston: Beacon Press, 2011.

Wendler, David, and Annette Rid. "Systematic review: The effect on surrogates of making treatment decisions for others." *Ann Intern Med* 154 (2011): 336–346.

Wilt, Timothy J., et al. "Systematic review: Comparative effectiveness and harms of treatments for clinically localized prostate cancer." *Ann Intern Med* 148 (2008): 435–448.

Wolf, Gary. "The data-driven life: Technology has made it feasible not only to measure our most basic habits but also to evaluate them: Does measuring what we eat or how much we sleep or how often we do the dishes change how we think about ourselves?" *New York Times Magazine*, May 2, 2010.

Woloshin, Steven, Lisa M. Schwartz, Jennifer Tremmel, and H. Gilbert Welch. "Direct-to-consumer advertisements for prescription drugs: What are Americans being sold?" *Lancet* 358 (2001): 1141–1146.

Woloshin, Steven, Lisa M. Schwartz, and H. Gilbert Welch. *Know Your Chances: Understanding Health Statistics.* Berkeley: University of California Press, 2008.

Zeelenberg, Marcel, et al. "Emotional reactions to the outcomes of decisions: The role of counterfactual thought in the experience of regret and disappointment." *Organizational Behavior and Human Decision Processes* 75 (1998): 117–141.

———. "The experience of regret and disappointment." *Cognition and Emotion* 12 (1998): 221–230.

———. "The inaction effect in the psychology of regret." *Journal of Personality and Social Psychology* 82 (2002): 314–327.

Zenz, Thorsten, et al. "From pathogenesis to treatment of chronic lymphocytic leukaemia." *Nature Reviews Cancer* 10 (2010): 37–50.

Index

Index

Index